MIND AND BODY

MIND AND BODY

PRIYA D. LAL

GYAN

GYAN PUBLISHING HOUSE

NEW DELHI-110 002

MIND AND BODY
(Biology, Psychology)

Rs. 450

ISBN : 81-212-0797-5

Published in 2002 in India by
Gyan Publishing House
5, Ansari Road, New Delhi-110002
Phones : 3261060, 3282060, Fax : (011) 3285914
E-Mail : gyanbook@del2.vsnl.net.in
Website: http:\\www.gyanbooks.com

Lasertypesetting by : Varsha Graphics, Delhi
Printed at : Mehra Offset Press, Delhi

Dedicated to
my father Late Dr. Hari Prakash Lal
and
my mother Late Mrs. Premlata Lal
whom I love so much
and
I am thankful to them for my present status

Contents

Preface

Medical science has discovered and proved that there is a link between the immune system and the central nervous system. Science is finding that there are many physiological connections between these two systems. This is occurring as scientists learn more about the hormones and neurotransmitters that brain cells use to communicate with each other and with the rest of the body.

This book is a guide to a new way of looking at life, a way proven to lead to higher levels of awareness and satisfaction. The way to understand these states of inner discovery is through discipline of mind and body. All methods of meditation and chanting can lead us to successful inner journey and self-discovery.

When a man begins to develop his senses, so that he may see a little more than everybody sees, a new and most fascinating world opens before him, and the *chakras* are among the first objects in that world to attract his attention. The word *chakra* is a Sanskrit word, and it signifies a wheel of life and death. There are seven *chakras* which situated in various systems of our body. Man can achieve great success in the path of self-advancement by establishing a relationship with the powers of *Chakras*. This relationship can only be achieved through the inner journey in our body via meditation and chanting. It inspires man towards righteous wisdom. An astral, conscious electric current flows constantly in a person who is able to establish relationship with *chakras* via Yoga. It mainly influences his mind, intellect, heart and inner self. When energized these *chakras* can convert a man into a superman. Energized *chakras* can turn fear to joy, frustration to fulfillment, and will make man beyond limitation of time and space. It can heal us and get rid of various chronic illnesses in our body.

This book is written for those persons who want happiness

and heavenly bliss. This book will serve the purpose of the entire humanity including Christians, Hindus, Buddhist and others. As Jesus said "The kingdom of heaven is the highest state attainable by man is within us. He hath set eternity in the heart of man. (Luke III 10-14)". Man stands between the visible and the invisible worlds. Our ordinary level of consciousness is not the highest form. To get at the inner experience we must abstract from the outer. We must develop our *chakras.*

This book will also satisfy those people who think that religion is insensitive to human ills and social crimes do not appeal to the modern man. This book does not deal with religion to bring inner peace. The book uses the same techniques that are used in science and medicines.

My book distinguishes from others because it makes the bridge between physiology, philosophy and science. Many scientists from both physical and biological backgrounds have tackled the question of consciousness by starting with the properties of the physical brain, and then trying to see how consciousness might be adjusted in the brain. Here I present a reverse strategy. The theory starts by examining consciousness itself. From there we are then able to see how any or all of the possible features of consciousness can affect our brain and body.

Many people have written about *chakras* but they deal only with describing different *chakras* and their power. Very little is said about how to develop the *chakras* to the fullest extent and virtually nothing is said about interactions and eliminations of diseases by *chakras*. I have dealt with each subject in detail. It covers in detail all the topics mentioned above. I have made it one of my highest priorities to explain any facts, phenomena, or concepts in terms readily accessible to the general reader.

As I was born in Gaya, a city in Bihar state of India where Buddha, founder of Buddhism got his "Nirvana", a state where one feels unity of all life, a country, where meditation and yoga are practised in every place and mind over body is considered to be the fundamental truth of Indian religions. The seed of mystical philosophy of India was germinated in my mind by my grandfather who was the President of Theosophical Society of the State of Bihar. I have been doing meditation since my childhood and sometime I feel I am flying in the air with lightness. I immigrated to the United States as Mathematician in 1971. Beside my professional job in the Department of Defence I am also involved in various philosophical and volunteer work of teaching mathematics during weekends. I have written many articles on philosophy which have been published in local newspapers. I have three Master degrees in M.Sc. in Mathematics, M.S. in Operation Research, and M.B.A. in Finance. My undergraduate degree consists of B.Sc. with Physics, Chemistry and Mathematics.

I am very greatful to Gyan Publishing House for having published my book in so short a time.

P.D. Lal

1

The Higher Body Element in Man: The Astral Connection

Mind and Body

Our body is full of wonders. We think we have only the physical body which has very limited capability. People who have developed intuition say that man has inner bodies, which, if properly developed, can become a powerhouse of immense nature. What are these bodies? The first one is the Physical body, second is the Astral body, third is the Lower Mental, fourth is the Higher Mental, fifth is the Causal, sixth is the Spiritual, and the seventh is called the *Atman* or self.

Man's Other Bodies

We learnt from the general observation that man has a physical body, which has seven different systems. We have bones, muscles, nerves, arteries, and organs of digestion, respiration and skin enclosing the entire body. This is only a chemical aspect of a man. This entire body is useless without the inner power that runs the body. This chemical body without the inner power is an inert body; it can't think or feel. It has no vitality, no intelligence; it lacks all the beautiful spiritual qualities which are common in human race.

Science tries to endow physical matter with super-physical qualities and powers. How are the higher powers contained in the physical body? Science is unable to explain these spiritual powers. They can only be able to analyze the body; genes, DNA, cells but they don't have any explanation why the genes receive heredity. They do not have any explanation how the life develops in the body. Science can't say why some people are born blind or some are blessed with high intelligence.

Theosophy tells the super-physical orders of matter, specialized for just those forces, and gives a logical, understandable answer that breaks through the impasse that science has reached. Science has found more than 100 elements in the physical world, but there are elements finer than physical elements which are found in man's other bodies, like, Astral, Mental, etc.

Theosophy tells us that there are subtler bodies that man possesses which function in co-operation with the physical body. Man has several subtler bodies, each makes its own contribution to the family of bodies.

All these invisible bodies interface each other and with the physical bodies.

The subtler bodies are invisible and can't be seen by ordinary eyes. Man can see all his subtler bodies by means of his third eye. For convenience, it will be necessary to show them separately, but they all interpenetrate. Each one has its own specific contribution to make a family of bodies. Many people have had out of body experience in which they have been out from their physical body and experience the minuteness of the subtler bodies and have returned back to their physical body and have written experiences. This kind of experience can only be had by means of deep meditation.

Just as the unseen parts of the physical body are seen by using a microscope to extend physical vision, similarly, the unseen super-physical bodies can be seen not by microscope but by those who, in the course of their life hastened evolutionary process by means of going into deep *samadhi*, through which they developed powerful sense organs which penetrate the super-physical bodies.

Another body we shall consider is the family of body which is a vital body. It surrounds the physical body. Any spiritual person can see the vital body which covers the aura of physical body. This vital body can be seen on the back of the head of people who are highly spiritual. This body is the source of power supply of the system. It absorbs energy from the sun and spreads it over the nerves. It provides forces and energies to the body and generates electricity, which flows inside the body and nervous system, and contributes to the overall vitality of the body, including the nervous system itself.

The chemical metabolism of the body is responsible for providing primarily maintenance of tissues, and generating heat for muscle contraction and expansion. This etheric body is linked to the chemical processes through the generation and movement of electricity in tissues and nerves.

Our main supply of vitality comes from the sun and is absorbed into the ethereal body through specialized etheric organs within it. This absorption of energy is emitted to the physical body and this energy when reach the physical body is called "*PRANA*". When the vitalizing activity is completed then vitality and *prana* are projected outward in straight line from the pores of the skin. Mr. Leadbeater describes it as "bluish white" and having the appearance of being striated.

Ten years later Dr. Walter B. Kilner, of St. Mary's Hospital, London, published a book entitled *A Human Aura* in which he described observations he made of the aura of ethereal body for diagnostic purposes. The ability to see this body was induced by the use of slides made from Dicyanin Dyes in a solution of alcohol. Such a result is possible because, it will be realized, ethereal substances when induced within the physical body can be trapped in the physical world and while they are in the physical world and they are, amenable to the physical laws.

The Astral Body

The second most important body is called Astral. It is a body of passions, desires and emotions. It resides in the centres of our sense organs—of sight, hearing, taste, smell and touch. So this body envelops all the nine gates of the body. As the astral body is made of matter of very fine texture as compared with the visible body, and has a great tensile strength, it changes slowly due to changes of passions and desires that are generated due to physical body intense activity. During a lifetime, while the physical body alters every moment the astral body alters slowly.

It has immense strength, and at the same time it possesses

elasticity permitting its extension to a considerable distance. It is flexible, plastic, extensible and strong. This body due to its flexibility can be extended and contracted due to the ebb and flow of passions and desires of the physical body. The matters of this astral body generate electrical and magnetic attractions in the physical body.

If the passions, desires and emotions are low and have a high density, their vibrations consequently are slow, and the colours of the astral body are dark, dull brown, dark reds and greens. Low vibrations of passions means that passions are full of material desires and ego. A person who have brown red astral body indicates is a greedy person; grey-green indicates deceit and cunning; brown astral body indicates selfishness; scarlet indicates anger; yellow round head indicates intelligence; grey-blue above head indicates primitive religious feeling; touches of deep rose color indicates beginning of love. A Green colour astral body indicates sympathy; blue astral body indicates a religious feeling. All the above colour have been discovered by Leadbeater by means of out of body experience.

For the educated and refined people the astral body has a reached high state of evolution. People who can go out of the physical body have found that there are seven subdivisions of an astral body. Each of the subdivision elasticity depends on the materiality and corresponding condition of matter. Each of these sub-planes interpenetrates the plane or sub-plane below it, due to these interpenetrating of bodies the flow of energy from one body to another has taken place easily. So that here at the surface of the earth all exist together in the space, although it is true that the higher varieties of matter extend further away from the physical earth than the lower.

All the seven planes of astral body are intermingled with each other. Consciousness of a person moves from one plane to another. Highly evolved person's consciousness easily move from different layers of astral body, whereas in a less developed person consciousness is inactive and remains in the lower level.

So when we speak of a man as rising from one plane or sub-plane to another, we do not think of him as necessarily moving in space at all, but rather as transferring his consciousness from one level to another gradually becoming unresponsive to the vibrations of one order of matter, and beginning instead to answer to those of a higher and refined order.

Matter of all astral sub-planes specially lower sub-planes which are similar to earth materials exist on the surface of the earth, but the astral planes are much larger than the physical, and extend some thousands of miles above its surface. Since the dense astral matter existed near the earth surface so they are affected by the earth gravitation. The law of gravitation operates on astral matter. So there is much intermingling due to gravitation of the earth. It is true that the higher we rise, the less of the denser matter we find. It is less dense because the gravitation of earth effect is reduced.

Sub-planes in the astral body can be divided into three main groups or classes. Density of astral planes is inversely related to higher numbers, i.e., higher the number the more dense it is, whereas lower the number the less dense. So these sub-planes are numbered from highest and least material downwards, we find that higher numbers are denser than lower numbers. 1, 2 and 3 forming one such class, and 4, 5, 6 another, while seventh stands alone. The difference between the matter of one of these classes and the next would be related to the difference between a solid and a liquid, while the difference between the matter of the subdivisions of a class would rather resemble that between two kinds of same dense material in the astral plane as on earth plane such as, steel and sand.

The life on 7, 6, 5, 4 are very similar to life on the earth without the physical body. While other group of planes are more rarefied and have less material.

If we look at something by astral senses, the physical objects look into true appearance. People who have developed their astral powers can perceive the object in an unbiased form whereas the physical eye is conditioned with the mind and we can't see the true image of an object. Thus experience will indicate that such vision approximates much more closely to true perception than does the physical sight. Looking from the astral plane, the sides of a glass cube would appear equal, as they really are, while looking from the physical plane we see the further side in perspective—that appears smaller than the nearer side, which is mere illusion. It is this characteristic of astral vision which has led some writers to describe it as sight in the fourth dimension. So the person with an astral vision can see the events in the future and mould his actions accordingly.

With our physical eye, we cannot detect minute particles of air. Our physical eyes' vision are limited and many atoms are only seen by a microscope. Again perception of the world by physical senses are possible sources of error. Matter is further complicated by the fact that this higher sight is cognizant to forms of matter which while still purely physical, are nevertheless invisible under ordinary conditions. Such, for example, are the particles composing the atmosphere, that all the various emanations which are always given out by everything that has life, and also four grades of still finer order of physical matter which, for want of more distinctive names, are usually described as etheric. We can see all these sub-particles through our astral eyes.

We must note that every physical body, which is made with material elements there, has a corresponding astral counterpart; this counterpart is a complex body composed with various kinds of astral matter. Take, for example, man's body which has corresponding astral materials. Similarly, animals also have their astral materials.

The head of the highly superior individuals who have spiritual manifestations is surrounded by a halo which is comprised of astral elements. The most brilliant aura seen of all perhaps, is astral, which includes that part of the aura which expresses by its vivid and ever changing flashes of colour the different desires which sweep across the man's mind from moment to moment. Take, for example, person who is in intense anger, his anger can be seen through his eye. Whereas in case of a person in a happy mood his eye will reflect the same.

One other point which deserves mention is in connection with the appearance of physical matter when looked upon through as astral plane, that is, the higher vision. This vision when fully developed, possesses the power of magnifying at will the minutest physical particle to desired size, as though by a microscope, though its magnifying power is enormously greater than that of any microscope ever made or ever likely to be made.

The ordinary atoms when seen by the astral eye appear to be much more complex in their nature than the science have ever known of. It opens the new knowledge and vistas needing more than a lifetime for examination. Through astral eyes one can see the orbits of revolving electrons, protons and neutrons and also have a glimpse of the anti-matter, which does not obey the laws of relativity.

It will be noted that these objects resemble the ordinarily objects of the physical world from the background to life on certain levels of the astral plane, yet so much more is seen of their real appearance and characteristics that the general effect differs widely from that with which we are familiar. For the sake of illustration take a rock as an example. When regarded with trained eye it is no mere inert mass of stone.

Seeing from the astral eye the appearance of stone will not be inert matter, but it appears as vibrating and pulsating energy which is constantly in motion. Through the astral eyes we can glimpse the whole of the physical matter of the rock whereas by physical eyes we can see only the small part of it; secondly, the vibrations of its physical matter has a corresponding astral part composed of various grades of astral matter, which are also moving in constant motion. Through the astral eyes one can see the vibrating life of a stone.

The Universal Divine life, which is active at each stage of life, has different manifestations and power at different stages of evolution. Universal divine life manifestations can be seen much more in man than in animals, vegetables, and minerals. For the sake of convenience each stage has its own name. We can see more universal motion of life in the trees and animals through our astral eyes. People can contribute in the science of DNA and cells by looking through astral eyes.

It is very difficult for us to grasp this reality which we cannot see with our physical naked eyes. It is difficult to accept the existence of the astral body when we can't sense the same by our senses. Science tells us that all life which is flowing in the world cannot be conceived by the physical senses. Our senses are limited. We cannot see the air that surrounds us. We can only feel the air when it is blowing. When this air becomes a hurricane it can throw down our strongest buildings. Clearly all about us there are potent forces which elude our partial and poor senses. It is error to assume that what we see is only the true reality.

We are, as it were, shut up in a conditioned body in which the senses are tiny windows. There are nine gates of a physical body and corresponding to these there are nine windows, which enable us to glimpse some thing outside. These gates always open from outside. There are nine guards, which include our ego and passions, they always push us out when our mind tries to enter inside. In many other directions we are entirely shut in, but clairvoyance sight opens for one or two additional windows, and so enlarges our prospect for the wider world of which we are quite ignorant.

It is important to see and grasp correctly the physical and astral world. Different bodies are connected through memory which reside in a brain. So in order to pass informations to different bodies one has to develop his memory and store the information in the memory. One has to carry the physical consciousness to astral plane then to mental plane without any break, and go back again to physical world.

Memory has a tendency to forget events, specially shorter events. In this exercise, if the memory is not developed then it is difficult to recollect all the information in our mind and some of the information are lost during the blank interval which separates our period of consciousness on various planes.

Most of us experience astral vibration when they are sleeping. At that time they are awake on the astral plane during the sleep of the physical body, since our mind is always indulged in physical passions so we are very rarely awake in the astral plane while we are sleeping. And yet, we are generally very seldom awake to the plane, and consequently we are conscious there very vaguely. Since, our experience in the astral plane is clouded with physical passions, we are completely unaware of the astral experience.

We are still wrapped up in our waking thoughts and our physical plane affairs, that we pay scarcely any attention to the world of intensely active astral body.

Our first step, then, is to shake off this habit of thought, and learn to see that new and beautiful world, so that we may be able intelligently to work in it. In our waking consciousness any recollection of astral planes are lost. We can remember the astral planes by developing our memory by *yoga*.

The person without any psychic development who floats about in his astral body during sleep never enters in a deep and calm flow of the astral currents. So he often wanders in a more or less unconscious condition. In deep sleep, the astral body almost invariably withdraws from the body, and hovers in the immediate neighborhood. In this condition people can experience a deep sense of peace and tranquility.

A person who is quite undeveloped, has the astral body as a sleep as their body. Never the undeveloped person never enters in an astral plane. In some cases, however, this astral vehicle is less lethargic, and floats about in various astral currents, occasionally recognizing other people in similar conditions, and meeting with experiences of all sorts, pleasant and unpleasant, the memory of which is totally confused.

All cultured people, belonging to the higher races of the world, have at the present time their astral senses fairly developed, so that, if they were sufficiently aroused to examine the realities which surround them during sleep, they would be able to observe them and learn much from them. But in majority of cases, they are not so aroused, and they spend most of their nights in a kind of thought which may have been uppermost in their minds when they fell asleep.

They have astral faculties, but they scarcely use them; they are certainly awake in an astral plane, and yet they are not least awake to the plane, and are consequently conscious of their surroundings only vaguely, if at all.

Premonitions, consist of, the sensing of the unseen presence and many allied experiences due to the activity of the astral body and its reaction on the physical body; People who have developed their astral body can enjoy premonitions, and can see the future from their astral eyes. They do not depend on chance and uncertainties. Their ever-increasing experience frequencies are merely the result of their evolution. In a few generations it will be so generally developed that it will become as familiar as the physical body. After death we live for some time in the astral world and in the astral body used during our life on the earth, and the more we learn to control and use it wisely now, the better for us after death.

A well developed body in the physical world can exist after death, and people can enjoy heavenly bliss whereas people whose body is vague remains in a hell fire.

The Mental Body

The mental body, is made of finer material than the astral, as the astral is finer than the physical. This body, answers by its vibrations to our changes of thought. Particles of this body are subtler than astral body. This is the body where thoughts are generated. Every change in thought makes vibration in our mental body, and this is transmitted by the astral to the physical. This causes activity in the nervous matter of our brains. This activity in the nervous cells causes many electrical and chemical changes in them, but it is the thought activity, which causes these, and not the changes, which produce thought. Thoughts are the first step in performing any action. Our thoughts are formed according to our past *karma*. Positive thinking and peaceful thoughts can produce successful results. You cannot do any action without interaction of thinking. The scientist first blueprints the research project in the mind then he makes it workable in the physical world.

The mental body, like the astral, varies much in different people; it is composed of coarser or the finer matter according to the needs of the more or less unfolded consciousness connected with it. In the educated, it is more active and well defined; in the undeveloped, it is cloudy and has dark colour. Its matter is drawn from the mental plane, and it is continuously active, for man thinks in his waking consciousness. Thoughts power is a force like electricity and gravitation. Physicists have proved that thought power is a subtler force which can be transmitted from one mind into another mind and produce good or bad effect depending upon the thought.

As this is the body in which long centuries will be passed in the heaven world, it is only rational to try to improve it as much as possible here.

The means are study thought, the exercise of good emotions, prayer and beneficent endeavours, and above all, regular and strenuous meditation. The using of these will mean a rapid evolution of the mental body, and an immense enrichment of the heavenly life.

Evil thoughts of all kinds befoul and injure the mental body and if these evil thoughts persisted it will result in veritable diseases and maiming of the mental body, incurable during the period of life. Evil and fearful thoughts produce depression and are a cause of heart attack and other dreadful diseases. Looking at the mental body of the primitive man we see little development as of now. Similarly, mental body of monkeys and other animals are very little developed. However, some yellow colour in the mental body at the top indicates a slight amount of mental ability of primitive man. Some improvement is shown in the average man and, in the man of high development advanced mental powers are evident. All the colours in it are much more refined and delicate and the yellow of his intellect is displayed in great strength, to which is added actual beauty of appearance.

Each of the bodies grows by use. The physical body grows through the exercise of its own faculties. So do the higher bodies. Use of abuse, action or neglect, will raise or lower the quality and responsiveness of the bodies. Mental body can be developed by meditation and chanting.

Illustrations of effect of depression on the mental body are shown in the sensitive plate. Dull grey bands begin to form around the body, which gradually transform into a kind of prison house of dejection if the condition is allowed to continue. This depression will cause blockage in the flow of blood through our veins and the person can get any deadly disease.

In the extreme cases if the man always has passionate thoughts then his astral body will be more gross and all the light colours of the body are obscured and the man becomes a virtual prisoner of its own Astral vehicle.

The effects of fear are somewhat akin to that of depression. But here, rather than showing as a steady deadening effect, fear will cause grey horizontal lines to vibrate with great agitation and almost obscure the normal colours of the body. Each such disturbance, however, will leave the body a little more prone to succumb to fear because of the kind of matter built into it.

Anger is another violent emotion and causes great havoc within astral and mental bodies. In the intense anger the colour of the astral and lower mind becomes red. These angry thoughts will block the ability of discrimination. Man cannot discriminate good or bad and when discrimination is lost then man performs heinous crimes.

The individual expressing such a murderous emotion, as this must have given way to anger many times before, otherwise the body could not produce such violent eruptions of malice and hatred. Knowing these facts, it is important to give heed to signs of danger and to overcome the difficulty before it becomes too powerful to be surmounted such that nature's drastic must intervene.

Note particularly that, it is not the spiritual man himself who gets angry, or feels depressed, or is fearful due to outer reactions of senses. When the nine senses control the mind then he fails to control his astral body and he becomes imbalanced. Careful analysis of the conditions of our consciousness at such a time will often, probably invariably, reveal that there is an inner voice, the voice of the self, which is vainly trying to be heard above the violent reactions of the body and desperately trying to control the body and to bring it back to condition of balance.

The Spiritual Body

We have a body which is the dwelling place of Super Consciousness, an image of God. According to Saint Paul "for in this body we groan, earnestly desiring to be clothed upon with our house which is from heaven". In *Bhagawat Gita,* Lord Krishna said that I am sitting in every body's heart as a Super Consciousness. Man's immortal bodies, where atoms are much more lighter and subtle than astral and mental bodies, build this heavenly house. This is the residing place of spirit, which is sitting in it through unending ages, through births and deaths.

The Spirit which is "the offspring of God" shares in his eternal life. This Spirit we call monad, because it is a unit, the very essence of Self-hood. It is existing all over the universe. Presence of this energy causes elliptical movement of the earth around the sun. Entire universe including galaxies are blessed with super consciousness presence. The brightness of the star and the emission of energy by the sun is the result of super consciousness direction.

The Monad, when he descends into matters in order to conquer and spiritualize it, and break down into three higher worlds—the super-spiritual, the spiritual and the intellectual.

All these bodies including spiritual are connected by a thread of energy called Buddhic. This thread of Buddhic energy connects spiritual, mental, astral and physical bodies.

These higher bodies exist in higher mind, by which the man deals with abstractions, which is "of the nature of knowledge", in which he knows truth by intuition, not reasoning, borrowing from the lower mind. Man can utilize the vast power of super consciousness by controlling the ego and let the higher mind control the lower mind.

When super consciousness directs the lower bodies to the path of progress will be smooth and the man is attracted in the path of evolution. The man in this body is called the ego, and when this body blends with the next above it is called spiritual ego, and begins to realize his own divinity.

It is by nature separative, being the instrument of individualization in order to give the necessary stability to the subtle spiritual body, which it is, blending. These are man's immortal bodies, subject neither to birth nor death; they give the continuous memory, which is the essence of individuality;

they are the treasure house of all that deserves immortality. They are the ever-lasting dwelling place of the spirit.

The *Atman* or Self is encased in the Spiritual body, the Spiritual body is encased within the Causal body, the Casual body is encased in the Higher Mental, the Higher Mental is encased in the Lower Mental, the Lower Mental is encased in the Astral, and the Astral is encased in Physical. So, our Physical body is the vehicle of our self or *Atman*.

The ordinary waking-consciousness of man is the consciousness working through the physical brain at a certain rate imposed by it, conditioned by all the conditions of that brain, limited by all its limitations, bulked by the varying obstructions it offers. This brain is conditioned by our previous *karma*. Intelligence of a brain does not always depend upon the past *karma*. If the previous *karma* of a person is bad and egoistic then the brain is conditioned by the previous passions of life. In this case, the brain is the greatest slayer of reality. If it is conditioned you cannot conceive the true image of reality. If you wear blue glasses every thing looks blue, but if you see through blue glasses a green tree that tree will appear black. At every moment the brain hinders its manifestations, while at the same time, it is on the physical plane it is only enabling instruments of manifestations.

When consciousness, turning its attention away from the external world, ignores the denser part of the physical brain, and uses only the etheric portions thereof, its manifestations at once change in character. In this case, the conditioning is not so much as in case with physical brain.

When it casts aside an ethereal garment, it begins roaming through an astral world at will, and receiving many impacts from the astral world. These impacts are either ignored or accepted according to one's stage of evolution. The perceptions of object of a person who has developed higher level of astral body will be quite different from the person's whose astral body is not developed.

Should it manifest itself to an outside observer—as it may happen in Trans conditions—its power of observation is superior to those it manifested when imprisoned in the physical brain.

When a person goes into a trance he will experience a heavenly bliss in which his consciousness becomes silent and its beauty will dazzle the observer. What is more is that the astral body, once it is thrown into a trance, will illicit the Bird of Heaven to show itself soaring into loftier regions, and its beauty will amaze the observer; its vibrations are more superior than physical and astral planes.

Most people have not developed the higher bodies so they are not in a position to appreciate any evidence of unity of consciousness which is working above the physical plane. However, its unity on the physical plane is being shown.

In order to understand the body we must first understand the amazing physical powers of the body which we unknowingly ignore every day.

2

Basic Units of the Body

There are four main levels in the human body. The smallest living units are called cells. There are about 75 to 100 trillion cells existing in our body. All these cells are divided into 100 different types. Millions of cells along with non-living material called matrix form tissues to perform some basic functions. The tissues in turn form organs to perform some related tasks.

Some cells look like columns, some like cubes, others like spheres. Red blood cells resemble saucers, other blood cells look like threads, cheek stones look like paving stones.

Although all cells have the capacity to produce, store and utilize energy, some of them do very specialized functions. Our heart cells perform different functions than liver cells. There is divisions of labour for millions of cells.

Each cell is enclosed within a membrane. A membrane resembles like a nucleus of an atom in which electrons and protons circle in an orbit. The nucleus of an atom where mass of an atom is concentrated is similar to the nucleus of a cell in which the cell's center of mass is enclosed (like a nucleus of an atom it acts like a control centre), and a cytoplasm where most of the cells work is done.

The membrane of a cell is a thin envelope which protects the cell from foreign invaders.

A membrane acts like a guard to the cells. It has special physical and chemical properties that allow it to recognize and interact with other cells and to decide what may leave or enter the cell.

Like a security guard the membrane thus stops the unwanted intruders. A typical normal cell obeys the stop and go signals, but cancer cells disobey the signals in an uncontrolled manner. It may be possible that unchecked defective cells in the cell membrane have something to do with the spread of cancer. Cancer cells are like criminals who disobey the guard.

The heart of the body is like a foreman in the production factory, which controls the chemical reaction of the cell in a controlled manner. It also pumps the blood throughout the body.

The nucleus of every cell contains a complete set of the body's map. Inside the nucleus of a cell there are 46 thread-like structures which are called the chromosomes. Each chromosome contains thousands of genes. Genes are the minute particles of a chromosome which are influenced by hereditary of parents. Without the nucleus the cell loses its ability to produce, and eventually dies.

The living matter outside the nucleus is called the cytoplasm. This watery gel cytoplasm has a specialized function of transporting, modifying and storing proteins to different destinations. It is like a department manager of a store. And also disposes wastes.

Where Does the Cell Get its Energy From?

Science says that cells take energy from a chemical compound called ATP (adenosine triphosphate). This chemical compound is present in every cell of the body.

These ATP are produced by food we eat. The actual work of generation of ATP goes on in the tiny structures of the cytoplasm called mitochondria—the cell's power plant.

Suppose ATP could be drained from our body and crystallized from 3500 calories of food, our cells could make a mound of white powder measuring 3 cubic feet. Now, suppose the chemical energy in the powder could be converted into electrical energy, there would be enough to power 1,500-100-watt light bulbs for a full minute.

How did the cell receive the power to convert the food into energy?

The Hindu Vedas say that the brain is the supreme electrical power house, with all the centres connected to one another and acting under the influence of the supreme center (mind). The mind discharges life current, or electricity, through these brain cells which, in turn, discharge electricity to different nerves which respectively carry motor impulses and sensations like touch, sight, smell, sexual impulse and others to our nine gates of body.

The electrical flow from the brain is the life of the organism; it is also called the *prana.* It controls the movement and is the electrical medium through which all our sensory reports reach the brain and cause thought reactions.

The Self, which controls mind if it wishes to shut out effectively the disturbing reports of bodily sensations, it must control and channelize the electrical flow through the nervous system as a whole to the seven main centers (which are discussed later). By this process it may give the outer and internal organs perfect rest.

In sleep, the electrical conductivity between the brain and the sensory organs is partially obstructed, so that ordinary sensations of sound, touch, and so forth, do not reach the brain.

However, because this inhibition is not complete, a sufficiently strong stimulus from within restores this elclectical conductivity inside the brain and it reports the activity to the brain, and a person remembers when he awakes up.

Yet, there is always, in sleep, a steady electrical flow into internal organs like the heart and lungs as well as other parts so that they keep on throbbing and working.

What is the Internal Environment of the Body ?

Each cell consists of a watery gel which is in our internal environment. It is called extracellular fluid, or ECF. It is so named because it lies outside the cell. One-third of the fluid is outside the cell, and two-thirds inside the cell. The extracellular fluid is constantly in motion everywhere in the body; all our cells are bathed in it. The cells actually live in it, in somewhat the same way as the sea creatures live in the ocean.

Our cells can grow in this internal environment provided it contains the right amounts of amino acids, fats, glucose, salts and oxygen.

How does the cell nucleus relate to chromosomes and genes?

A primer to heredity must begin with the cell. As said above, the cell contains a nucleus, which is the control center. Inside the nucleus there are 46 thread-like structures known as chromosomes and contained in each chromosome are thousands of genes. Chromosomes and genes are made of DNA (deoxyriboundeic acid) which transfers the hereditary material from generation to generation.

All these hereditary messages are stored in our universal molecule, which imprints all the traits of the physical, astral, mental, and casual bodies. Science cannot explain why the person who is, say, not very intelligent is sometimes blessed with a highly intelligent son, or why a highly intelligent person often ends up having an idiot son. Intelligence transfers take place due to the store of energies from previous lives.

How is the Body Organized?

There are ten systems in the body by which the entire body functions. The ten systems are:

Nervous System

This includes the brain, spinal cord, nerves, and also the eyes and the ears.

The nervous system controls all the activities and functions of our internal organs-even our thoughts and emotions. The brain is composed of three principal divisions : first is the cerebrum, the second is cerebellum and the third is brain stem. Intelligence, learning, and judgement are said to reside in the cerebrum which is the first sector of the brain. The cerebellum maintains equilibrium and controls muscular activities. Whereas the brain stem controls hunger, sleep, and sexual behavior.

How the brain sends messages?

The brain uses two kinds of powers—electrical and

chemical. Electricital power moves the message from one end of a long nerve cell to another. Chemical power moves the message from one cell to another in a more complicated process because cells are not directly linked. The messages in the brain are transported by one gap to another by neuro-transmitter which pour out of the end of the cell just as the messages approach the gap.

The electrical power that has brought the message so far now shuts down, and the neuro-transmitter takes the message abroad and moves it across the channel to the next cell along the route. Then the electricity comes on again, and the whole process is repeated until the message reaches its destination.

We do not see by our eye alone, but rather with our eyes and brains together. The eyes pick up impressions from the outside world and send messages about the world to the brain for interpretation. If one's primary visual cortex were removed or destroyed they would be blind, even though there is nothing wrong with their eyes.

The Endocrine System

This system controls and coordinates the body functions such as the development of sexual characteristics.

The nervous system and endocrine system are sister systems in communicating and controlling the body elements.

The nervous system sends the messages by electro-chemical impulses, which travel quickly to muscles and glands whereas the endocrine system sends the messages by means of hormones which act like a chemical messenger in transmitting the messages to cells. The hormones also help maintain a constant environment inside the body, adjusting the amount of salt and water in our tissues, and sugar in our bodies.

Diabeties is caused by the insufficient amounts of secretions of hormones. It is associated with a disturbance in the normal insulin mechanism.

Glands of Endocrine System

Most of the glands in our body's fall into two categories. The first category is exocrine and the second endocrine. Exocrine glands are the outside glands that secrete their products outside the body or into a cavity. Examples are the salivary and sweat glands. Endocrine glands reside inside the body and empty their products inside the body. They have no ducts; instead, they secrete the products directly inside the body. Glands of these types are pituitary, thyroid and adrenal.

There are some glands that perform both the functions of exocrine and endocrine glands. These types of glands are called pancreas glands.

The Pineal Glands and the Soul

This gland is the place where mind and body meet. This is called a mystery gland and is shaped like a cone. Scientists agree that it serves as a kind of internal clock. It responds indirectly to lights. Messages of how much light is reflecting are transmitted to this gland by the eye. As the daylight fades to darkness the pineal glands start secreting hormones called melatonin. As the day advances this gland slows down the secretion of melatonin. This gland is responsible for afffecting seasonal changes in our body.

How many Hormones are there?

Not long ago there were about 40 hormones in our body, but now it is believed that there are 100 or more.

Since blood travels through every part of the body, and is also pumped to the hormones some people might think that each hormone is affecting all the organs of the body, but the hormones generally affect only certain parts of the body and transmit its messages to a particular cell or target cells. Each hormone has an affinity for some special cells. That particular hormone can only affect that cell.

In a way, hormones work like keys in a lock. Only a certain key which fits in a certain lock can open that lock. Similarly, particular hormones can deliver its messages to particular cells and receptors. Today hormones can inhibit as well as stimulate the body's processes. Hormones can unlock particular cells and when the cells are open one can experience the energy of that cell.

Hormones act as a switch on genes. Sometimes they do shut off their supply which cause shut down of energy and sometimes they resume their supply resulting in flow of energy in the genes. They sometimes slow down the cells functions and sometimes speed up the cell functions. Sometimes these hormones are controlled by the mood of a person. Depressed person will release energy which will dilute the unlocking powers of hormones.

Some hormones produce short-lived effects within seconds of their release, while others act more slowly and create long lasting effects.

Pituitary and Master Glands

The pituitary gland was once believed to be the control gland of the body. It is the gland the which is directly linked with the brain, and through the brain as a master it controls the various parts of the body. The hypothalamus is an essential link between the brain and the pituitary. In reality, the hypothalamus, which is in endocrine system, feeds back the hormones in a controlled way. For example, the hypothalamus releases hormones stored in the pituitary—among them oxytocin is vital in child birth and nursing. Its release also turns on hormones from the anterior pituitary, which stimulates secretions by other endocrine glands.

How our Brains and our Bodies Talk to Each Other?

The brain and bodies talk to each other through the hypothalamus. The hypothalamus monitors information about the body states and it is the main coordinator of activities in the nervous system and those in the endocrine system. The hypothalamus acts like a computer which has connection with brain and receives energy from the brain and transmits it to every part of the body.

When messages from the brain travel through the hypothalamus, and that hypothalamus transfers those messages to the other organ that organ feels the sensation and gives the good vibration of those sensations. It also gives awareness of what is outside our system, such as levels of circulating hormones and the concentration of the nutrients in the body.

Hinduism explained the same doctrine in a similar way in which the hypothalamus is like a *prana*. The brain and body talk to each other via vital energy called *prana* or vitality. This vital force was unknown to Western scientists. *Prana* is a Sanskrit word, derived from the word *prana*, which means to breathe, move, and live. Thus, it is called the life-breath or life-energy. As in Hindu thought, there is only one life that is connecting to all the creatures that is called the *Prana*. It has been proved by science that all genes of all creatures are similar in 98 per cent and differ only in 2 per cent. So life energy or *prana* is essential for all the creatures of the world.

In Western scientific terms, this energy is called vitality. As a coordinating and connecting energy it binds the physical molecules of the body and fills them with an everlasting energy. All the molecules are bathed with this energy. Without *prana* there could not be any life on this planet. Without *prana* the body could be a collection of independent cells without any action. *Prana* links and connects these into a one complex unit of life. *Prana* is absorbed by all living organisms, a sufficient supply of it seeming to be the necessity of their existence. The sun supplies *Prana* energy. Sun energy along with air is converted into vitality energy is called *prana*.

It is the life for living animals and plants. It should be inhaled in moderate quantities. Too much presence of it in the nervous system may lead to disease and death, just as too little leads to exhaustion and ultimately death.

H.P. Blavastsky compares *Prana*, the active power producing all vital phenomena, to oxygen, as without oxygen there could be no combustion. Oxygen is the life giving gas, the active chemical agent in all organic life. On the physical plane, *prana* builds up all minerals, and is the controlling agent in the chemico-physiological changes in protoplasm, which leads to the differentiation and building of the various tissues of the bodies of plants, animals, and men.

Similarly, *prana* acts on an astral body. The astral *prana* blending with physical *prana* creates nerve-matter, which is fundamentally the cell, and which gives the power to feel pleasure and pain. The cells develop into fibres, as a result of thought; the *prana* pulsates along those fibres, which are composed of physical, astral and mental *prana*.

The Secret Doctrine speaks of *prana* as the invisible or fiery lives which supplies the microbes to elephants with vital energy, thus enabling them to build up their life from the size of the smallest infusoria, to that of an elephant, lion, tiger or camel and man. By the manifestations of *prana*, the speechless appears as the speaker. Nose which is inactive starts smelling, tongue which looks like a sleeping rubber starts tasting foods.

The whole doctrine of constructive vitality in the universe, and in man is thus summed up in *prana*.

Paracelsus thus referred to *prana* "The whole of the Microcosm is potentially contained in the Liquor Vitae, a nerve fluid in which is contained the nature, quality, character, and essence of all beings."

The ancient Aryans sang that Surya "hiding behind his yogi, robes his head that no one could see."

The nerve centre, which are controlled by the *prana*, direct the energy to the dense body. The nine gates of the dense body start bubbling with the energy and these nine gates then act outwards with different passions. So *prana*, the controlling energy, which acts through the nerve centres, making the food-sheet obedient, and fashioning it for the purpose which the I, seated in the higher intelligence, demands.

The physical contacts are transmitted inward by *prana* to the astral body and these vibrations are subtle than the outward vibrations. These inward vibrations are acute, sharp, keen, specific, and overall being quite different from the heavy, diffused sensations deriving from the cells themselves. It is by means of the astral body that *prana* runs along the nerves of the body and thus enables them to act not only as the carriers of external impacts but also of motor forces, originating from within.

So the *prana* acts like a power of the brain. The currents of *prana* activate the brain, which contains trillions of cells interconnected by nerve wires. Without this the brain will be a dead brain.

The sitting place of *prana* in the brain is the mind through which all the senses are controlled. There is an allegorical story in the Veda which illustrates this. It said that all the eyes, ears, nose, tongue, and brain started fighting about the supremacy of their power. They wanted to settle the dispute by mediation through the Lord Brahma. The Lord said that any senses would be superior and most powerful only if it withdraws from man and the man dies.

When the eyes withdraw from the man, the man becomes a blind man. There are many blind men in the world so the eye is not the most powerful sense. Similarly, when the ears withdraw from the man the man becomes a deaf man, and can still survive those crises of his life.

When the brain withdraws from the man, the man becomes brainless and he is still not dead. When the tongue becomes actionless the man can survive by taking liquids. Now comes the *prana*, when *prana* withdraws, the entire body is dead including all the senses. So, *prana* is the supreme of all senses.

The Respiratory System

The description of the *prana* is very similar to the respiratory system described by doctors working in the field. This is called the breath of life. Every day we breathe in and out 5,000 gallons of air. This respiration accomplishes two things-it supplies the body with oxygen, and takes the carbon dioxide out of the body. The oxygen is the life supporting gas whereas carbon dioxide is inhaled by the plants and emits oxygen. The rate and depth of respiration vary, depending on how quickly the body uses up oxygen and how fast it accumulates carbon dioxide. This depends on the activity level. The lungs perform most of the respiratory functions. The lungs are a pair of not-quite-identical, cone shaped organs that lie within the chest cavity. When we inhale, the air—one-fifth of which is oxygen—enters the air sacs of lungs, and then it pumps the oxygen to the blood in the capillaries. Some of the entering oxygen is dissolved in the blood, but most of it combines chemically with haemoglobin, and is carried by it to the tissues. When the capillary blood reaches the body it goes to regions that need it.

At the same time, the blood picks up the carbon dioxide produced by cells, and returns it to the outside by the exhaling process. So inhaling oxygen is entered in lungs and exhaling carbondioxide is pumped out.

Pulmonary veins which carry oxygenated blood from the lungs to the heart are located behind the heart, whereas Pulmonary Arteries carry blood laden with carbon dioxide from the heart to lungs.

The Circulatory System

One thing is clear that our heart looks very much like the pear-shaped object shown on Valentine's Day greeting cards.

The heart, according to some experts, never rests. The heart never ceases to beat when life lasts, it continues to contract and relax over and over again. From this it may be inferred that the heart never rests.

In cases of sensed danger, tension, conflict, anger, or depression adrenaline pours into our bloodstream, elevating blood pressure, causing the heart to race fast. Doctors cite these physiological changes as evidence for their belief that emotional stress can harm the heart, as the high blood pressure and rapid heartbeat accompanying it may have a harmful effect on our body. The high blood pressure can damage the valves of the heart, and the person will die due to stroke.

The heart consists of two pumps, each with two chambers. The right side of the heart receives blood partly depleted of oxygen from the body's outlying areas and pumps it into lungs where it is replenished with life giving oxygen. The left side receives this oxygenated blood from the lungs and sends it to the rest of the body.

The left side of the heart is more muscular than the right because it has more work to do. The left side of the heart pumps blood at higher pressure to the most distant parts of the body. So, it is more muscular. The heart itself has three layers of specialized tissue. The outer one is epicardium—a thin, shiny membrane. Next comes the thick heart muscle called the myocardium, which performs the main work of the heart. Finally, there is another smooth, shiny membrane, the endocardium, which lines the cavities of the heart.

According to Vedas, the Self or Atman, which is called the Supreme Soul or God resides in this heart. This Self which prevails in the entire universe is the unconscious force existing in the heart. Astral, mental and casual body sheets further encircle this Self. This Self is the silent witness of the entire activity of our life. It is also a witness to all other activities of our previous life experiences. In it, many of our past horrifying experiences are absorbed from our previous or present lives. Sometimes people having a split personality or other emotional breakdown syndrome are the result of expressions of those hidden emotions to outside body.

According to some doctors, the only way those syndromes can be eliminated is by releasing those hidden thoughts out of one's unconscious memories. These depressing hidden thoughts can be released by doing meditation.

According to Vedas the Self is a subtle form. This Self which is called Super Self is immortal, it is unlimited, it is imperceptible. The essence of that form which is subtle, immortal, unlimited, and imperceptible is the following principal : this is the Self and essence of our living body. The living body and lower mind are mortal. It is mortal because its desires are temporary and binding. People who get rid of all desires become immortal.

This refers to the subtle body of self. As sun emerges in the morning and suddenly illumines all around, so does Self, as it emerges from the unmanifested, bring to light all things?

The Self or Super Self, according to the Veda, should be realized, this super self is not heard of, but it is reflected when it is awakened up or when meditated upon. By the realization of the Self alone one can get a *nirvana* state of ultimate unity of life? In that case there is a perfect silence.

The Self is beyond hunger and thirst, grief and delusion, decrepitude and death. Realizing this very Self, people give up the desire for sons, for wealth, and for world and take up a wandering mendicant's life.

The Digestive System

This system controls the hunger and thirst that emerges

in the body at constant intervals of time. We don't need a stomach to feel hungry. People whose stomachs are removed still feel hungry. The brain which controls the levels of amino acid, glucose, fat and other substances of the blood sends out the signal to us that we need food. Stomach does not create hunger, but brain is the creator of all the hunger and thirst. People who are diabetic always feel hungry and thirsty. This is due to high level of glucose in the blood.

Similarly, we are loosing water all the time through the skin, the lungs, and the function of the kidneys. The brain receives the signal that we are thirsty from our blood. Insufficient water in the body reduces the volume of blood, and, therefore, the blood pressure.

The digestive system operates like an assembly line in reverse, taking whole foods and breaking them down into their chemical components. It is like a food processor in which all the vegetables and fruits are channelled into the chamber where they are churned, mixed and come out in liquid form. Similarly, the food we eat is broken down by digestive juices into small, absorbable nutrients that generate the energy required to maintain life, replace the cells that are constantly dying, and keep it functioning. It replaces the dying cells with new young cells.

Importance of Saliva

Saliva breaks down starches into sugar. This sugar is the important element for maintaining our glucose level. Low or high glucose level is bad for health. It moistens it so that it can be chewed and mixed into a ball. The third functicn of the Saliva is to keep the mouth healthy.

Role of the Tongue

The tongue plays an important role in speaking and in eating. It gives us pleasure in eating.

There are four primary tastes—salty, sour, sweet and bitter. These come from the chemical compounds in foods that we eat. Extreme of each taste is bad for health. Moderate amount of salty, sour, sweet and bitter are acceptable to our tongue and body.

Taste is highly individual. This means that people not only like different foods but that the same foods may produce different food sensations in different people. And then too each person's saliva has its own tastes. These food sensations are due to different types of genes in different bodies.

If, for example, our saliva has low sodium content, foods containing a given amount of salt tastes saltier to you than a person whose saliva is high in sodium that food does not appear saltier to him. Saliva can become moderate doing exercise, whereas dehydration, and illness can affect the composition of saliva from moderate to extreme.

Fluids pass rapidly out of the stomach but solid foods need time to disintegrate. Our digestive system breaks down the food and absorbs all the juices and expels all undigesitve food from our system via stool.

The hydrochloric acid which the stomach secretes is corrosive enough to dissolve a razor blade or annihilate living cells.

The Liver : A Chemical Factory

The liver does 500-odd functions. It includes the manufacturing of glycogen, and stabilizing the blood sugar level. It builds enzymes, processes digested fats and proteins, remove waste products, manufactures bile and cholesterol and are an important source of heat. People whose liver is not processing properly are likely to get various diseases. No wonder the amazingly versatile liver is frequently likened to a chemical processing plant.

The liver is a kind of magician. It can turn sugars and fats into protein. It also makes sugar out of protein. The liver serves as the receiving center and storage area for most of the glucose absorbed from the small intestine.

The Reproductive System

White in colour and shaped like an egg, each testicle is divided into 250 to 400 lobules that contain the tiny semi-niferous tubules in which the sperms are produced. The sperm plays an important part in the reproduction process.

Pair of testicles or testes which lie inside the abdominal cavity in the pouch is called the scrotum, it produces the sperm, which fertilize the female eggs.

Each sperm contains 23 chromosomes, or half of the man's genetic code. If and when sperm unites with an ovum, which also carries 23 chromosomes, the result is a fertilized egg containing 46 chromosomes—all the hereditary information needed to create a human being. To ensure the survival of the human race, nature is lavish with reproductive cells. When a girl is born, her ovaries contain about 2 million primordial ova, or potential eggs. A person whose sperm is not powerful to fertilize cannot have a child. Similarly, women whose ovum is unable to conceive with sperm will be childless. In either case artificial simmentation procedure is used for childbirth.

3

The Force Center of *Chakra*

The *Chakra* in Sanskrit (mother of Indian languages) means a wheel. The Buddhists call it a wheel of life and death. It is also called a wheel of righteousness and truth. Through the literal meaning it is called a wheel of the law. This *chakra* moves and rotates by the force of law of *karma*. For the people who have built up too many passions in the law of *karma* this wheel rotate faster, whereas for saintly people it moves at a moderate speed.

Here the word *chakra* is used to denote wheel like vortices, which circle our etheric double.

Man's physical body is changing all the time. Medical science has discovered that every cell of our body is undergoing transformation every minute. This physical body needs three types of energy. These energies are derived from food, water and air.

Energy from food and water are important for digestion and the maintenance of the body. Energy from air is for breathing and vitality. This vitality mix with sun energy becomes "PRANA". This *prana* is a cause of all the life energy of a body. This *prana* when directed in a proper way energizes the body and *chakras*.

There are seven centers of the body. All these centers are rotating like a wheel. Energy flowing from top is flowing from one center to another.

This force breaks down into seven component forces. Without this energy the physical body could not exist. Therefore this energy is in operation in every person. In an ordinary person these forces are sluggish and slow. In a more evolved man they appear glowing and pulsating with living light. The *chakras* can be energized by energy derived from food, water and air. Sexual desire, which is byproduct of food, water and thought, can be channeled from sexual organ to the upper portions of *chakras* by means of meditation.

Most of the divine energy which activates the *chakras*, enters from the head and this divine energy which pours into each center act on a right angle. This divine energy acts like a magnet. When the magnet is thrust into an induction coil it produces a current of electricity which flows at right angles to the axis of the magnet.

Similarly, this divine energy produces energy at right angles to the axis of *chakra*.

Any person who has some inner power can see the wheel like the saucer on the back of the head of some highly spiritual man. When quite undeveloped for the ordinary man, it looks like a 2-inch diameter circle of dull and sunshine. But in a highly spiritual man, they are seen as blazing, coruscating whirlpools, much increased in size, and resembling a small sun. See the pictures of Jesus, Buddha, or Gandhi. On back of their heads there is a small shining wheel noticed in the pictures.

These *chakras* can be divided into three sections—lower, middle and upper. The lower section is called physiological, the personal and spiritual. The first two centers which are in the lower group receives the energy from physical level—one being the serpent fire which comes from the earth, and the other energy comes from the sun. This serpent fire resembles with intense sexual desire. This second energy is called vitality. The *chakras* 3, 4 and 5, which are makers of personality, receive the energy as follows. Number 3 *chakra* receives energy from lower astral body, number 4 chakra receives energy from higher astral body and number 5 gets the energy from lower mental mind. All these centers seem to feed certain ganglia in the body. A person who receives energy from lower astral body seems to be more passionate and strong in desires. A person who receives energy from higher astral body is more moderate and spiritual.

Centers 6 and 7 stand apart from the rest, being connected

with the pituitary body and the pineal gland respectively, and come into action only when certain amount of spiritual development has taken place. This only happens when mind of a person is without any ego and is calm and quiet and without any desires.

The seven centers, which are present in every human being, are illustrated as follows :

1. Root or Basic Chakra. In Sanskrit, it is called *Muldhara*. It is situated at the base of a spine, or in the Reproductive System as described in the first chapter. It is the most active *chakra* for all creatures. It takes energies from the food and earthly minerals and causes a lot of sexual desires and vitality. It is like a red flaming cross burning like a fire, and energy radiates from it. This is also called serpent fire. The power of this center can be channeled to other centers by means of Yoga.

This *chakra* is a primary force that radiates out in four spokes, like a cross. One quadrant of the cross is red, another is orange, a third one is red, and the last one is orange. It means that the four quadrants are alternately red and orange. Sometimes this becomes a radiating hot cross that starts emitting vitality to other centers and also receiving energy from the spleen center.

2. Spleen Chakra. In Sanskrit it is called *Savadhisthana*. It is situated in the neighbourhood of the generative organ or over the spleen, around the lower parts of the digestive system. This *chakra* receives the vitality from the sun. This center has six petals or sub-divisions. After getting the vitality from the sun it breaks down the sunrays into different colours like a prism. Each of the six sub-divisions represents red, orange, yellow, green, blue and violet. After breaking into different colours it pours out the vitality to different *chakra*.

This second center is called the spleenic center, which after receiving vitality from the sun breaks down the sun rays into red, orange, yellow, green, blue and violet. Each of these colours then radiates to different centers and energises that center. This *chakra* is a main source of sending energy to different centers and is radiant, glowing and sun like.

3. Navel or Umbilical Chakra. In Sanskrit it is called *Manipura.* It is situated at the navel, over the solar plexus and one can locate this *chakra* at the upper portion of the digestive system. This chakra has ten wheels or sub-divisions. When in motion its vibrations are more than the spleen chakra which has six sub-divisions. It receives the red and green colour from spleen *chakra*. Each ten sub-divisions are either red or green. This powerful *chakra* also receives its primary energy from the sun and breaks down into ten directions, corresponding to the ten undulations or petals.

Its main colours are the various shades of red and green. After receiving green colour from the spleen center, the rays also flood the abdomen, liver, kidneys, intestines and the digestive system.

This center is closely associated with feelings and emotions of various kinds. This is mostly influenced by the astral body.

4. Heart or Cardiac Chakra. In Sanskrit, it is called *Anahata*. It is situated in the circulatory system of the body. It is an important vital place of the body. From the heart the blood is pumped throughout the body via veins. It has twelve sub-divisions. It glows in golden colour. It receives the yellow and orange colour from the spleen chakra.

This awakening center transmits the yellow colour to different parts of the body, including the brain. Since the heart pumps blood to the entire body, along with the blood the colour yellow produces vitality in various parts of the body. When this colour reaches the brain it produces a power of love and kindness.

The corresponding astral center, when awakened, endows a man with the power to comprehend and sympathize with others.

5. Throat or Laryngeal Chakra. In Sanskrit it is called *Vishuddha*. It is situated in front of the throat, its ideal location is the respiratory system in the body. It has sixteen sub-divisions or petals. It receives the blue and green colours from the spleen *chakra*. Blue and green predominate alternately in this section.

This *chakra*, the fifth, has sixteen spokes, and therefore, sixteen petals or divisions. It receives the violet ray from the spleen *chakra*. This ray then breaks down into light blue and violet blue; light blue travels into the throat and dark blue goes inside the brain.

The light blue gives energy inside the throat, and emits strength and elasticity to the vocal chords of a great singer or speaker.

The dark blue expends itself in the lower central parts of the brain, while the violet floods the upper part and appears to give special vigour to the *chakra* at the top of the head, diffusing itself chiefly through the 960 petals of the outer part of the center. Thought and emotion of a high spiritual type seem to depend largely upon the violet ray.

6. Bow or Frontal Chakra. In Sanskrit it is called *Ajna*. It is located in the space between the eyebrows, and this *chakra* is situated in the endocrine system which is described in the previous chapter.

It has 96 sub-divisions or petals. The certain jump from 16 to 96 is indicative that we are dealing with higher level of *chakra*. This *chakra*, when energized, emits energy six times more than heart *chakra*. It, sub-division is filled with rose colour, mix with yellow.

These 96 sub-divisions represent complexity and multiplicity of the human personality.

The sixth center, the frontal isolated between the eyebrows. It is divided into two petals. Each of these two petals are divided into 48 sub-petals. Thus, the sixth *chakra* has in total ninety-six petals.

This *chakra*, when awakened, causes a man to begin to see objects, and to have various sorts of waking visions of places or people. When fully developed it brings about *clairvoyance*.

7. Crown or Coronal Chakra. In Sanskrit it is called *Sahasrara*. It is situated on the top of the head and prosaic location is in the nervous system of the body. It controls the brain, spinal cord, and nerves including the eyes and ears. It has 972 sub-divisions or petals. When this *chakra* is energized it starts vibrating with almost great force and rapidity. Its colour is violet. This *chakra* is last to be awakened. In the beginning it has an it size as other *chakra*. As man moves in the path of spiritual advancement the size of this *chakra* starts increasing and then covers the whole head. In the oriental pictures of god and goddess the head is radiating like a sun on the back of a head. In a highly developed man, this *chakra* pours out splendour and glory which makes for him a radiant crown. This radiance of this *chakra* can be obtained with long practice of yoga and meditation. When man is awakened he finds the unity of life in this *chakra*.

All these wheels are perpetually rotating, and into a hub or open mouth of each force from the higher world, it is always flowing—a manifestation of the life stream issuing from the Sun, which is called a primary force.

This force is seven-fold in nature. As a ray of light can be broken into seven primary colours of light, so this force can be broken into seven components.

All these forces operate through all the centers, without which there could not be a body. Therefore the centers are in operation in every one, although the radiance varies in individuals. In an undeveloped man its forces act in a sluggish manner, but in a highly developed man it is glowing and pulsating with living light, so that an enormously greater amount of energy passes through them.

Each of these secondary forces that generate in the *chakras* radiate like a light, but it does not travel in a straight line. Instead, it travels in a wave, like undulated vibrations, containing several sub-waves within it. Each of these sub-waves contain different wavelengths of smaller size than the primary wave. The wavelengths are infinitesimal, and probably thousands of them are included in one of the undulations. As the forces rush round in the vortex, these oscillations of different sizes, cross one another like flowers blowing from a stem. One can thus see why Hindus compare the *chakras* to flowers originating from a steam.

These *chakras* are naturally divided into three groups—the lower, the middle and the higher. They are seen as the physiological, the personal, and spiritual. The Root *chakra* and Spleen *chakra* are lower *chakras*, and while one is connected with earthly forces while the other one gets vitality from the sun. The *chakras* three, four and five are middle *chakras* and arc generally associated with personality.

The Navel *chakra* gets the energy from the lower astral body whereas the Heart *chakra* is energized by higher astral forces, which are devotion, charity, love, and sometimes laziness. The forces of the lower mind originate in the Throat *chakra*. If the vibrations of the lower mind are pure this *chakra* will emanate good vibrations; otherwise it is inactive.

Centers 6 and 7 stand apart from the rest, being connectec with the pituitary gland and the pineal gland respectively, anc come into action only when a certain amount of spiritua development has taken place.

Although the likeness to petals is caused by the same force: flowing around the center, alternately, over and under th various spokes, these spokes differ in character. That is, becaus the in rushing forces are subdivided into its component parts o qualities, and therefore each spoke radiates a specialize influence of its own, even though the variations may be slight The secondary force in passing each spoke, is to some exten modified by its influence and therefore changes a little in it hue. Some of these shades of colour may indicate a form of forc that is helpful to the growth of the moral quality of man.

The following quotation, which was written by Indian Philosopher Krishnamurthi, is wholly applicable in regards tc the *chakras*.

"In oneself lies the whole world, and if you know how to look and learn, then the door is there and the key is in your hand. Nobody on earth can give you either that key or the door to open, except yourself."

Let us examine the *chakras* in detail.

The seventh center is the coronal at the top of the head.

When stirred into full activity, it becomes one of the most powerful *chakras* of the body. It contains all different types of hues, but is predominantly violet. The number of the radiations of the primary force in the outer circle is one hundred and sixty. In addition to this, it has a feature which is possessed by none of the other *chakras*; a sort of subsidiary central whirlpool of gleaming white flushed with gold in its heart—a minor activity which has twelve undulations of its own.

This center receives in its outer portion the violet ray that passes through the throat center, while in its central portion it receives the yellow ray from the heart center. This *chakra* is attached with the pituitary gland. It also communicates with the pineal gland, which directly communicates with the lower mental spheres. This explains the emphasis sometimes laid on the development of the pineal gland.

The awakening of the etheric center enables a man through it to leave the physical body in full consciousness, and also to re-enter it without the usual break.

Medical science has discovered and shown that there is a link between the immune system and the central nervous system. As a result, science is finding that there are many physiological connections between these two systems. This is occurring as scientists learn more about the hormones and neuro-transmitter that brain cells use to communicate with each other and with the rest of the body.

Immune Basic

The immune system is the body's means of defense against infectious diseases and cancer. It has two primary tasks : to distinguish between "self" and "non-self", it destroys, inactivates, or eliminates foreign substances that are identified as non-self.

The two major arms of this protective complex are the humoral and the cellular immune systems. In the humoral system, white blood cells produce antibodies and proteins that are key to the body's defense bacteria and viruses in body fluids against the foreign invaders.

Antibodies do not carry out the cellular immune response, but various immune system cells carry it out. One of them, which carries out the responses, is called the T-lymphocytes, which help organize the overall immune response, and which engulf and dissolve invading organisms. Another type of immune system cells are natural killer cells, which defend against virus-infected cells and cancer by attacking them and destroying them.

Billions of B-cells are on guard the body at all times, and each one is geared to recognize a single specific kind of invader, or antigen. So billion B-cells can recognize billions of different antigens. When an antigen appears in the bloodstream, it is "caught" by a receptor on the surface of the appropriate B-cells.

Next, the B-cells engulf and surround the antigen and expose part of the antigen on its surface, where it can get help by a helper T-cell which then attacks the invader and destroys them.

The T-cells attach to the B-cell and release chemicals that stimulate the B-cells and convert it into an antibody factory that is called the plasma cell. The plasma cell then multiplies in the cells and pumps out those produced millions of identical antibodies into the bloodstream where they encounter the invading antigen.

Antibodies can render invaders harmless in a number of ways. For example, they can latch onto toxic substances produced by bacteria, inactivating the toxins.

Chakras and the Immune System

The above example shows that God has given us such a powerful inner body which always protects us from foreign invaders. But are we taking advantage of such a powerful gift from God? No, many people become victims of stress which weaken their immune system. Thus, they become victims of invading antigens and get infected with cancer, AIDS, and other deadly diseases.

If the *Chakras* are fully developed they will energize the body and secrete the chemicals, which will boost the power of the body and protect us from deadly diseases like AIDS, cancer, and other diseases.

The elevated *chakras* will help to maintain the helper/

suppressor cell ratio in optimum balance. People with AIDS and other immuno-deficiency diseases have low ratios; if those people raise their helper ratio by help of *chakras* then they eliminate those diseases and make a strong auto-immune system, characterized by an overactive immune system.

Coronary heart disease is America's number one killer. Stress seems to play a more subtle, long-term role in the overall development of coronary heart disease. Stress and eating red meat, eggs causes problem in the heart.

There is growing evidence that learning to become less hostile and by increasing peace of mind and suppressing anger and developing stronger connecting networks of heart can improve the prognosis for many people with coronary disease such that they survive the heart attack.

People who are in stress develop high blood pressure. This is a result of raising adrenaline, which triggers the movement of fat from the body's fat stores into blood streams. This adrenaline raises the levels of cholesterol, which then accumulates in plaques. Whereas people who do meditation transmit billions of neuro-transmitters which dissolve all the fatty deposit of the tissues. This can save and prolong our lives and make us happy and stress-free.

Hostility can be neutralized with a commitment to change, to learn to control our reactions and behaviour. Research also shows that support groups who believe in *chakras* can improve the prognosis for heart patients and it is reasonable to believe that strong social support for changing habit could help healthy people prevent heart disease as well.

4

Forces Acting in the *Chakras*

Kundalini

Energy of the *Kundalini* comes from the sun and part from the earth. It is different from *Prana* as it cannot be converted into another form of energy. *Kundalini* exists in all planes. It also appears to have seven layers or degree of forces. Each layer has different degree of power. The terrific power of the Kundalini comes from the earth. It belongs to the red glowing fire from the earth.

The earth gets the power from the sun and emits the stored energy to the *Kundalini*. The fire that comes from below is much more material, and has a burning sensation like the fire of red-hot iron. This is a tremendous force that descends deeper and deeper into matter, and moves upward slowly like a serpent fire.

When the *Kundalini* is awakened at the astral level, in the center corresponding to the base of the spine center, it moves to the second center, near the navel, and vivifies it, thereby awakening in the astral body the feeling of passion.

Kundalini then passes to the third, fourth (heart), fifth (throat), sixth (eyebrows) and seventh (top of the head) spleen centers in turn, awakening in each the various powers. When it reached on the top of the head it energizes the whole body and cleans the body from all diseases.

The Marriage of the Forces

As the stems of all the *chakras* look like a flower-bell and its root starts from the spinal cord, this force naturally flows down those streams and pushes the flower-bells, where it meets the incoming stream force of divine life. The pressure set up by that encounter causes the radiation of the mingled forces horizontally along the spokes of the *chakra*.

The divine force is called a masculine force, and the downward descending force is called *Kundalini*, which is generally feminine in character. These two forces revolve in opposite directions and meet at the point, which is called the marriage of the two forces.

The combination of these two forces form the compound force and this becomes powerful like a magnet and the person who has developed this magnetic force will attract people from the outside. This magnetic force will transmit the energy to the other person and another person will feel attracted by that force.

It also intensifies the plexuses and hormones, which are situated in the neighbourhood of several *chakras*; it flows along all the nerves of the body, and is principally responsible for keeping up its temperature up and diseases down.

Anatomists describe two nervous systems—one is called "Cerebro-spinal" and another is called "Sympathetic". Cerebro spinal is connected with the brain. It gets energized and intensified from brain it pumps energy to all main points of the body including *chakras*. The brain gets the energy from the *prana*. Whereas the sympathetic system consists of two cords which run in the spine. From this sympathetic system a network of nerves emerge and formed nodes, which appear like relay stations for releasing energies to the *chakras*. In addition, we have the third group called the "Vagus" nerve, which descends from the medulla oblongata and also pumps energy to different plexuses and other systems.

The intermingling of these forces resemble like a *Shiva-linga* which represents a creative power of the world. Shiva according to Hindus is an energy, which changes form. This *linga* extend upwards and descends downwards into the earth. This *linga* shows the circular flow of energy similar to the flow of energy in our body. This clearly shows that ancient Hindus had knowledge of occult. So the *Shivalinga* represents the flow of energy in our body.

Cells of Consciousness

If the brain were cut apart to reveal its smallest working components then the smallest part would look like a tiny factory forty thousandths of a millimeter in diameter. These components are called neurons. These neurons are the different components of a tiny factory.

Neurons can be seen under a microscope. They look like dark blotches with thin branches emanating from them. We cannot see neurons from our naked eye. They can only be seen through microscope.

Andrew Huxley developed a model for describing how the living nerve cells could generate electrical signals.

All the neurons are found to contain dendrites, which is called tree in the Greek and resembles it and its branches emanating out into progressively thinner processes.

These dendrites are the main receiving area for inputs from brain to neurons. The axon conducts signals from the cell body to make contact with dendrites of the next cell. Although almost all neurons have dendrites, a cell body, and an axon, their overall shapes vary enormously. So the energy passes from one dendrite to another through an axon and this process energizes the entire body.

The chemical activity of the brain is transformed into electrical energy. Then this electrical energy excites the neurons. Neurons differ in other cells of the body as they emit electrical energy. These electrical signals are the result of chemical activity of four types of ions (chloride, calcium, sodium, and potassium), amounting to a net imbalance of charge across the outer wall of the series, which is called the membrane.

The imbalance of these charges generates a potential difference, which causes a voltage drop and results in an electrical flow to other neurons. Hence, it is possible to create electrical signals which are the building blocks of brain activity. Some of these signals are synchronized with the emitting signals and some are unsynchronized. Some of the synchronized signals become powerful and generate power inside the body.

Whereas consciousness that arises from the brain triggers the chemical reaction and is the real master of the brain activities, the basic components through which consciousness performs action are chemical ions and neurons. Consciousness is not the by-product of neurons, but it is the controller of brain activity. If we assume the brain to be as a computer then mind or consciousness is the computer programmer who controls the computer.

Not knowing the connection between a nugget of gold and solidity, glitterness and brightness as non-subjective phenomena will lead to delusion. Similarly, it is of critical importance to distinguish between identifying what particular elements or events in the brain make up the mind and subsequent questions of how the mind actually emerges from them. It is important to know how brain controls all the nine gates of the body. Brain and mind are different. From mind consciousness emerges and that consciousness controls the brain.

Center of Consciousness

Modern science has also described different centers of sub-consciousness. All these centers of sub-consciousness reside on different levels of *chakra* and get energy according to Descartes from a pineal gland—a small region deep in the center of the brain, the seat of the mind. The brain is like a command station that effectively directs signal and enables and keeps an enduring and consistent mental state to survive the ebb and flow of consciousness. This brain is the permanent home of the mind.

As soon as different brain regions were identified and categorized a very serious question arose : Does the brain work as a whole where all the regions interchange information freely? Or it works in parts? Sometimes it works as a whole and sometimes it works in parts; specially it works as a whole in case of damage of a brain and transfers energy to damaged parts. It tries to overcome the damaged brain regions, which leads to specific deficits like Parkinsons disease the inability to move. It is noted that when the brain is damaged, the neurons of other areas rush to compensate the loss by rushing towards the damaged parts. Similarly, certain brain regions are closely associated with the function of vision; it is interesting to note brain is not functioning cannot see in spite of good eyes. There are as many as thirty such areas located throughout the brain that are associated with the vision.

In building up an integrated view of the brain from its gross parts it is found that each region has a certain function such as pleasure, conscience and motor control.

On the origins and relations of the sympathetic and cerebro-spinal systems Dr Annie Beasant wrote :

"Let us see how the building of the nervous system by vibratory impulses begins from the astral plane of our body and is carried on further to other parts. We find a minute group of nerve cells and tiny processes connecting them are responsible for transfer for energy to other parts of a body. This is formed by the action of a center which has previously appeared in the astral body- an aggregation of astral matter arranged to form a center for receiving and responding to impulses from outside."

These centers are pulsating to and from the center and pass energy to other planes. From the astral center vibrations pass to etheric bodies, causing little etheric whirlpools which draw particles of denser physical matter and then energizes the physical, centers which form a nerve cell, and then a group of nerve cells.

These physical centers receiving vibrations from the outside send impulses to the astral plane and rebound back and become a more effective force. The force then controls and energizes the vital organs—the heart, the lungs, and digestive tract and root *chakra*.

Then, it slowly energizes and develops the cerebro-spinal system which is closely connected in the lower workings of *chakras* with the sympathetic system, and becomes gradually more and more dominant in those *chakras*, while it also becomes, in its most important development, the normal organ for the expression of the waking-consciousness. This energy rising from astral plane now resides in the brain and the brain controls all the organs of the body by this energy.

So this cerebro-spinal system is built up by impulses originating in the mental, not in the astral plane; though the mental plane gets the energy from the astral plane. So cerebro-spinal is only indirectly related to astral through the sympathetic system built up from the astral.

5

The Dynamic and Psychic Forces Present in Nature

Vitality

Vitality is a dynamic force present in nature which revitalizes itself by sun rays and radiates into our bodies thus energizing our atoms. The effect of this varies. We sometimes feel cheerful and sometimes peaceful or spiritual. Science has discovered that every atom consists of electrons, protons, and neutrons. Each atom consists of several orbits like the solar system. In each orbit revolve the electrons or protons. The nucleus of the atom consists of neutrons because it has no charge. The revolving electrons, or protons, on the outer orbit determine the negativity or positivity property of an atom.

Science has proved that each orbit of an atom consists of space, and electrons and protons only occupy a tiny position in the atom. More than 3/4" area is empty and filled with some type of gaseous fluid like ether. This vitality enters in an atom through these ethereal parts and then passes the energy to the physical portion of an atom and the energy then passes from one atom to another atom and this vitality manifests itself in all our bodies—physical, astral, mental and casual.

However, we are concerned for the moment with its appearance in the lowest, that is, in the physical and its interaction with the gaseous fluid floating around interspace of orbits. This immensely increases their activity, and makes them animated and glowing. Since, we are presently in the physical world so interaction of vitality in the physical world is important for us.

We must not confuse this force with electricity, though it, in some ways, resembles it. It also differs from light or heat. Electricity, light and heat are denser forms of energies whereas vitality is the more subtle form of energy.

Though the vitality differs from those forces, when it enters in an atom from the outside or inside it causes oscillation of the atom as a whole—an oscillation, which is enormous as compared with that of the atom.

When vitality enters and absorbs in, the atom wells up in that way then within an atom it endows it with an additional life, and gives it, a power of attraction, so that it immediately draws around it, six other atoms, which it arranges in a definite form, thus making a sub-atomic compound called the hyper meta proton element.

Psychic Forces

This force, called the psychic force, is also called the spiritual force and it enters in higher *chakras*.

These forces can be trapped from outside by opening our minds by eliminating the ignorance and pride from our mind. This psychic force is present in the space and our mind is prepared to receive it. Like TV pictures waves are present in the space and when we look on the TV we receive the picture.

The first two centers of lower *chakras* exhibit none of these characteristics, but the navel *chakra* and others higher in the body are affected by this physic energy and in turn affect the human consciousness.

Psychics and Thought Forces

The third force behind primary vitality, and the *kundalini* is the psychic force. This force enters from the higher centers of a body, and this affects the human consciousness.

There are two main views accounting for these phenomena. One holds that everything is consciousness whereas the other holds everything to be form. The latter ignores the fact that form can only exist by virtue of life ensouling it. The form and the life are no different than matter and the spirit. The vehicle and the consciousness it contains are inseparable. Without consciousness form can't exist. A philosophy, which tries to explain everything by the forms, ignoring the consciousness, is ultimately lacking as an adequate explanation for phenomena. All phenomena in the physical world are the reflection of neumena of consciousness of the spiritual world.

However, a philosophy which tries to explain everything by the life forces, ignoring the forms, will not be very successful. For, it will find itself trapped by surrounding walls, which it cannot surmount. Just as you cannot see the power of electricity without electric bulb, same way you cannot grasp the power of consciousness without form.

The Self as "knower" has as its characteristic function of the mirroring within himself of the non-self. A sensitive plate receives a ray of light and changes the frequency of the light due to its ability to condition. Similarly, the Self receives a ray of image fully conditioned by the mind and can't perceive the true picture. If the Self is conditioned by theories, dogmas, beliefs then it transmits those conditioning to any image our mind received and we cannot see the true image of the object.

Hence the mind, which is the vehicle of the Self as knower, has been compared to the mirror in which images are seen on it. If the mirror is clean then we see the true image; otherwise we see the blurred image.

We do not know the things themselves, but only the effects produced by them in our consciousness. The mind, in its knowledge of the outer universe, knows only the illusive images and not the things themselves. Mind is said to be the greatest creator of illusion if it is conditioned and it is our best interest to slay the conditioning of mind.

However, it may be asked, as to how things must always be? This brings us to the vital distinction between the consciousness and the matter in which the consciousness is working with. By this, we can find an answer to that natural question which involves seeing the true image. True image can only be achieved by a calm and quiet mind.

When the consciousness, by a long evolutionary process, has developed the power to reproduce within itself all that exists outside it then the envelope of matter in which it has been working falls away. The consciousness, that is, knowledge then identifies itself with all the Selves amidst which it has been evolving, and sees nothing but the matter connected alike with all its selves. By the sameness of nature perfect knowledge is attained and the self realizes that marvellous state where the identity perishes not and memory is not lost, but where separation finds its ending, and knower, knowing, and knowledge is one. In this case consciousness and Self becomes one.

Motion and Consciousness

Life is motion. Consciousness is motion. And all motion affecting matter is vibration. The one, the all, we think of changelessness, either as absolute motion or motionless. When change of space is taking place in succession it is called motion. In this type of motion matter looks separated. All the motion is relative. When the motion is slow matter looks separated. When motion increases then matter becomes united.

When the one becomes the many, then motion arises. The essence of matter is separateness, as that of spirit is unity. When the twain appears in the one, it is like what we see happen with cream and milk. Absolute motion is a spirit. In absolute motion—the presence of every moving unit at every point of space at every point of time—is identical with the rest of everything. In that time of motion everything appears as one, and that is called spirit.

Spirit is like an infinite motion and matter is like a slow motion. Each spirit is enclosed in different bodies of various grade elements and is further enclosed inside the physical body of man. Each spirit is connected via vibratory thought to another spirit. An outside spirit receives the motion of thought if its own thought is in unison with the spirit it received the thought from. If the other thought is same vibration as ours then it energizes our thought power. This is one way of communicating with spirit level.

This phenomenon consequently causes a powerful force of thought generated by individual thoughts. If the receiver spirit thoughts are different than the sender spirits, this will not produce a perfect reproduction. Other thought power in this case will not produce powerful effect.

The sequence of vibratory actions is often seen in nature. A flame is a center of vibratory activity in ether, which is called heat. These vibrations, or heat waves, impinge the surrounding ether into like waves and make other ether in motion and when these bundles of waves strike a piece of iron nearby and pass heat to the iron piece, the iron particles vibrate causing the iron to become hot and a source of heat on its own.

Similarly, a series of vibrations pass from one spirit to another and all beings are inter-linked by this network of consciousness.

Matter of different densities surrounds us and we name the motions in it both by their densities and by how they affect ourselves. This is attested to by the different respective organs of our gross and subtle bodies. We name lights that are certain vibrations which affect our eyes. Certain vibrations are called sound which affect our ears, and the mind receives vibrations through the brain and interprets it accordingly. Some different densities of waves called smell are received by the nose and we thus get the sensation of smell. Seeing occurs when the light—ether is thrown into waves from an object to our eye; thinking occurs when the thought ether is thrown into waves between an object and our mind. So seeing, hearing, smelling, tasting and thinking are all controlled by the brain.

The mind is the result of past thinking, and is constantly being modified by present thinking. We get certain vibrations from our previous life thoughts, generated by us in a previous life, and stored in a universal atom. Our conditioning of thinking is the result of our past life habits and *karma*. We can change future by changing our thought-pattern.

It is thus that we have made these processes that we cannot change save slowly. We cannot transcend it by an effort of the will; we can't cast it aside, nor instantaneously remove its imperfections. All the results of our past thinking are present with us as mind, and each mind has its own rate of vibration due to our past conditions of mind, its own range of vibration due to our past life habits, and is in a state of perpetual motion, offering an ever-changing series of pictures. Every impression coming to us from outside is made on an already active sphere, and the mass of existing vibrations are modified by our conditioned mind and we cannot grasp the tı ue picture.

The resultant is not, therefore, an accurate reproduction of the new vibrations, but a combination of it with the vibrations already proceeding due to which the true picture is distorted. The influence of the mind as a medium by which the knower views the external world is very similar to the influence of a coloured glass on the colours of objects seen through it. Take for example, if we see an object through red glass the object looks red, although the object is not red.

It is in the superficial and obvious sense that the mind is called the "creator of illusion". It presents us only with distorted images, a combination of itself and the external object. These distorted images are images of appearances not of realities; shadows of shadows are all that it gives us. This illusion is caused by its own nature.

We cannot modify others but we can greatly modify ourselves. This we can do by greatly influencing our receptive capacity. If we increase the power of our reception we can transmit powerful thought forces outside as well as inside. When we develop the power of the mind, then our thoughts become like a white light, which contains the seven colours of the rainbow.

As this white light passes through our body, it will energize our other centers of the body by the strength of the colour of that center force. We may measure our approach to the whiteness by our power of response to the most diverse characters. If the finer vibrations generated from the outside and impacting one's mind are in same vibration with that mind, then it will generate a rapid and pure vibration in that mind and affect the subtle grades of one's mind substance. Our mind will fill with subtle energy. The coarser grades of our minds are not affected. When finer grade thoughts travel in our mind, they will go throughout the heavier grade mind particles and those particles will be replaced with finer grade particles. Similarly, base and evil thoughts draw into the mental body the coarser materials suitable for their own expression. These materials then repel and drive out the finer kinds. So when the people having an evil thought they become more depressed and sometimes commit suicide.

Thus, these vibrations of consciousness are ever shaking out one kind of matter and building in another. There is constant influx and exchange of thoughts due to our past conditions of thinking. It also follows, as a necessary consequence, that the kind of matter we have built into our mental bodies in the past, will effect our power of responding to the thoughts which now reach us from the outside. If our mental bodies are composed of fine materials, coarse and evil thoughts will meet no response, and hence can inflict no injury; so people who are in higher level of thinking always enjoy happiness and good health. Something, then, in the building and evolution of our minds may be done from the outside, but most must result from the activities of our own consciousness. For, we are our own builders and fashion our own minds for ourselves.

Many people like to read, but how one grasps what they are reading depends on their own thought power. If one reads a book with full concentration, he can grasp it well. But if our thought power is weak, our understanding of the subject will not be good. Unless a man takes up his thoughts and works on it himself, its value to him will be small and passing. This is also analogous to eating. Food will fill the stomach, but the meal is useless to the body unless it is digested and assimilated. So also reading may fill the mind, but unless there is thought, there is no assimilation of what is read, and the mind does not grow.

We can read five minutes and test what we have remembered for, we can discover the weaknesses of our thinking power. It is better to find our own weaknesses than to imagine oneself strong when one is feeble. If we concentrate on reading material and not thinking elsewhere we can grasp the subject well. Students who made high grade is all due to their concentration at the time of study.

The realization of the weaknesses of the wandering of the mind can be had by noticing feelings of heat, confusion and fatigue which comes on the brain after a prolonged effort to follow out a difficult line of thought. Wandering C. W. Leadbeter said thoughts are like energy, occupying a place in space.

Thoughts on the same subject and of the same character tend to accumulate; and they form a circle. The thoughts about the same matter are attracted to such a center and go to increase their size and influence. A thinker may be attracted toward a center and in turn influenced by it; and this is one of the reasons why people think in-groups like sheep. It is much easier for a man of lazy mentality to accept a readymade thought from someone else than to go through the mental labour of considering the various aspects of a subject and arriving at a decision for himself.

Thought flies like lightning through a subtle matter of the mental plane. So the thoughts of millions of people on certain subjects may easily gather together in one spot, and yet be accessible and attractive to every thinker on the subject. So people who do healing can operate in a group. Concentrated thoughts of so many people travel like a powerful force and help in healing.

To illustrate this, consider somebody filled with fear. The vibration of fear radiated from the mind of a body will attract any fear clouds that happen to be in that vicinity. If a man can control his fear then the extra rush of fear will rebound and leave the body. In this case the man is not hurt by fearful thoughts. But if a man cannot overcome the fear the extra onrush of fear will increase the fear more and more. The person will soon discharge the fear energy on the *chakras* and the fear will become a panic, in which the person may loose control of himself, and may rush blindly into any kind of danger. In the same way, one who loses his temper attracts clouds of anger, and becomes a victim of an in-rush of feelings which will change his feelings into intense fury like a fire which might lead him to commit murder by an irresistible impulse, almost without knowing it. Similarly, a man who is in depression may be drowned into a permanent depression by many other depressed thoughts around him. Or, one who allows himself to be obsessed by animalistic desires of sex, may become a monster of lust, and may become a rapist under the influence of those thoughts. Similarly, a man who has good thoughts in mind will attract more good thoughts from outside and he will evolve in an accelerating pace.

All such undesirable currents reach a man through the navel *chakra*. Whereas clouds of love and emotions evolve from the heart.

According to Dr Annie Besant, desire has two main expressions : the desire to attract, and the desire to repel. The desire of attraction will impart energy of attraction that will lead to further contact with that object. It will act like a magnet and attract other minds with powerful force of attraction whereas the desire to repel will drive one away from that object. The emotion which is of the nature of attraction, attracts objects to each other by pleasure, is the integrating energy of the universe which binds the world together. This energy which is in the form of emotion is called love. Emotions, which are the nature of repulsion, driving the objects apart, are the disintegrating energy in the universe.

These are the two stems from the root desires, and all the branches of emotion may be traced back to one of these twins.

Love seeks to draw to itself to the attractive object, the desire of love binds. Its ties are indeed more lasting, more complicated, and are composed of more numerous and delicate threads interwoven into greater complexity. The force of love attracts other person whereas the force of hatred repels the other person. If the thread of love is broken by hatred then that thread will never become one. It will have a knought in the middle.

And, hate seeks to drive from itself the repellent object, it is like a repulsive force from which we flee due to its unattractiveness and repulsion. Love and hate are the elaborated and thought infused forms of simple desires to possess and to shun. Love opens the heart whereas hatred closes the heart.

Love looking downwards is benevolence. People who are rich become benevolent and give money to the poor. Love looking upwards is reverence. Reverence is seen in the love between student and teacher. The normal relations between husband

and wife, between brother and sister are love between equals. Common characteristics of love between equals are the desire for mutual help.

Thus, we have benevolence, desire for mutual help, and reverence as the three main divisions of love-emotion, and under these all love emotions may be classified.

Similarly, hate for lower level people gets converted into scorn, hate for higher level people is turned into fear, this happens in the relation between boss and employee; and hate among equals becomes anger, disrespect, revenge, and violence. So hate among equals results in injury, killing, and other unlawful activity.

Vitality and Magnetism

Vitality is the energy that originates from the base *chakra* and circles around all the body and keeps a constant mixture of etheric parts of matter along the blood through the arteries and veins. This vitality energy is originated through the *kundalni.* Oxygen, which we inhale along with the etheric current, produces vitality. This vitality becomes strong if the force of etheric thought from the base *chakra* emits strong emotions. The particles of the etheric parts of a man's body are constantly changing. If the thought force is weak then vitality will be weak.

Medical science says that our blood cells keep changing as a result of the changing of etheric particles. The etheric particles are changing due to the food we eat or the air we breathe, as each of these particles contains the etheric matter. All these blood cells are constantly changing. In eight years all the blood cells are changed.

These etheric matters are concentrated on the etheric parts of the body. The etheric porus particles of a body are thrown out of a body like gaseous matter.

This is the reason if two persons talking with each other, and who are close together in their thoughts, can absorb much of the physical emanations of the other.

When one person mesmerizes another, either by magnetism or by thought power, he can push his own thought power in the mind of the other person. What is more is that the thought of the subject is replaced by the operator's thought and he acts at the will of the operator.

As the brain is the center of this nervous circulation, it brings that part of the subject's body, which is affected, under the manipulator's brain instead of the victim's. Thus the latter feels what the mesmerizer wishes him to feel.

If the man who is mesmerizing is trying to aid a diseased person, he can pour strength to the man by focusing his own thought power onto him. However, if the magnetizer's fail to give the mind is not pure then he might full impact to the mesmerizing.

Nevertheless, a man who is pure in thought and filled with the earnest desire to help his fellowmen may also do so by mesmerism in order to relieve suffering in the other person. Pouring the vitality fluid, the etheric fluid or a combination of both can do this. The pouring of energy from the outside will greatly benefit a patient who has emptied his own energy. This is one of the principles of healing.

The Mesmerist may renew such a patient's stock by pouring some of his own upon his quivering nerves, and hence produce a rapid recovery. Take the example of a man whose digestion is lost and he administers some tablets to increase it. Just as a man who is unable to produce specialized products for him may still absorb what another has already prepared, one can gain strength to make an effort to resume the normal actions of the etheric sphere on the organs. The etheric energy focused on an another person will produce an etheric bubble on another person's body and it will burst into divine energy.

Just as a man may pour out magnetism by an effort of will, so may he withdraw it by an effort? In dealing with a headache, he would probably lay his hands upon the forehead of the patient. He is pouring out the powerful magnetism from his body to his brain.

He is to first be a very careful and strong willed person so that he will not draw the bad and ill-thoughts of the other person, the result of which would be absorbing the headache of the other person and beginning to suffer himself.

6

Importance of Relaxation and Meditation

How to Develop *Chakras*

The first and foremost technique of developing inner powers is relaxation; this means throwing out all your stresses and emotions. Doctors at Harvard Medical School have said that by relaxation techniques the consumption of oxygen in the body is lowered. This is similar to sleep and relaxation responses bringing a decrease in oxygen consumption. The body's metabolic rate, an overall measure of biochemical activity, is reflected in the amount of oxygen consumed. Oxygen consumption drops significantly in meditators when they switch from simply resting to meditating and rises when they stop meditating. This decrease of oxygen consumption slows down the aging process, lowers the blood pressure as well as the pulse rate. In order to develop our *chakras* we should try to relax.

How to Relax?

Relaxation does not come through worry. Relaxation comes through tranquility of mind. A person who is working but thinking he is not working and a person who is not working thinking he is working that type of person mind can relax and he is not binded by the action. Simple method of relaxation is : every evening sit down on a warm and comfortable sofa; let no other person or telephone disturb you. Recognize your egos and bad thoughts, and release those bad thoughts. Releasing of bad thoughts is simply relaxing you; and you might fall sleep. You can also feel relaxed if you tune your breath.

Our stomach will move gently as we breathe in and out. Imagine that with each exhale you are releasing tension and you are reaching in a deep state of relaxation. Now, inhale the air and hold it down for one minute and then exhale assuming you are releasing tension.

This will help you in recognizing your personal self and tensions, and also helps us to release tension and feel relaxed. In this relaxation technique one might fall asleep. This helps us in sleeping better.

Worry our Worst Enemy: For many people life is a burden with worries. To quote an example, Brinda was worried about whether she was doing her job right, whether she would be promoted, whether others would recognize her abilities or ignore them. She was also worried about her boy friend. She was always thinking that her boy friend Mike is dating another girl.

It is important to know why some people are always worrying. Researchers have found that some people have genetic defects due to which they worry. It is also widely believed by experts in the field that experiences in childhood affect our tendency to worry.

Though Birenda was born with defective genes due to which she was worrying, but this did not mean that she could not change.

If you recognize yourself and even some of our worries then you can change this pattern and your worries can be controlled. The wavering mind full of worries is like a turbulent river which is wasting all the energy, but if that river is tamed by engineers then that same turbulent water will produce electricity and many houses will get light.

How to get rid of Worries: Sometime our life is full of trivial things. We worry about what we eat in the evening, how we will earn more money. When we fall in the waves of worry then one should raise these questions with oneself: "How important this worry is? How much this worry is going to affect our life—We can measure the impact of worry on long range of five years or ten years; we will then find that how trivial our worries are. Brinda found that asking herself "whether it will matter taken at all in five years time?" She found that most of the worries are short period worries. This helps her in disentangling the important from the unimportant things on the list.

When we worry think, "just how much worry is this worth". Our resources are limited our time is limited. Each day we are approaching the deathbed. It is easy that we can put too much of our limited resources in the wrong things. You need more energy for more important things. If you have persistent worry in your mind then ask question about yourself "is there anything I can do right now?" If you can do any thing then do it and stop worrying. If that worry is beyond your power then also stop worrying and channelized your energy to positive thinking. You can get rid of worries by imagination, by putting them out by sending waves of tranquil thoughts, which will blow out the worries. If you get rid of worry then your mind and body will be full of energy and vitality. The first step of reviving the *chakras* is to get rid of worries.

Build the wide wall around the worry if that worry is important for your life. If you think how to resolve it then think with a cool mind' only then will you be able to resolve the worry. And when worry is solved then that will turn into more constructive energy.

It is said that worries will age more on people than work. Work does not hurt the mind but the mental process, known as worry, definitely injures it. After constant worrying, our nervous system becomes exhausted and irritable. Worry is the process of repeating the same train of thought again and again, having no result or solution.

Perhaps the best way to get rid of a "worry" is to produce another, of an exactly opposite character.

Let, then, a person, who is suffering from worry, give three to four minutes in the morning, on rising, and generate some noble thought. Think that "The self is peace"; " I am the self"; "the self is undying, unchanging, fearless, free from all modifications."

He will then realize how mistakenly he regard worries. His slowly mixing with the higher self will bring in peace and enfold him, such that the mental energy will flow naturally into this channel, and worry will fly out like smoke.

Another method of getting rid of worry is ceasing to think

when you are alone. When we are thinking our mind is in constant action, and this useless thinking will harm our health. When work of thought is over we should stop thinking, and should not allow thoughts to drift our mind like a wave in the sea drifts the boat away. Owner of a machine does not allow the machine to run when there is no production. But we are running our priceless machinery—mind—aimlessly, without having useful result.

Constant worrying, constant vibrations in mind; constant vibration means constant waste. Exhaustion and premature decay result from this useless expenditure of energy, and a man may prevent from decay mental body and brain by stopping to think. It is true that "ceasing to think" is by no means an easy achievement. Perhaps it is even more difficult than thinking. It should be done slowly till the habit is established for not thinking. When you are attacked by waves of thoughts try to drop some thoughts by turning the attention away from those thoughts. It is just like turning away each intruder; if need be, imagine a void, as a step towards a silence. Practice on these lines. Your thoughts will become more and more intelligible and, peace and calmness will prevail in the mind.

Another way of silencing the mind and getting rid of worries is to change the thoughts. Constant thinking on one subject will create more problems; so changing the thinking pattern will help in reducing worries. The extraordinary freshness and youthfulness of thought in old age will fill the mind with bubbling energy and he will feel some youth-like energy. A man needs change of exercise in thought as well as in body, else he may suffer from mental cramp.

Peace of mind through expansion of our selves is important step in this direction. When we think about ourselves all the time and always want to satisfy our unfulfilled desires then we are in constant state of tension and peace of mind will be far away. All our troubles arise from thinking of us ourselves separated units, and then revolving on our own mental axes, thinking only of our separate interest, joys and sorrows.

Peace is not to be found in the continual seeking for the gratification of the separated self but it can be achieved by renouncing the separated self, and uniting all the self into one.

Desire for spiritual progress is of great value so long as we can control our lower self. We can free ourselves from lower desires by sticking to longing for spiritual growth. We are the Self, and therefore the joys and sorrows of others are ours as much as theirs. As the *Gita* said that "He attained peace, into whom all desires flow as rivers flow into the ocean, which is filled with water but remaineth unmoved". All the waves of the ocean started on the outer shore whereas the depth of the ocean remains calm. Similarly, our outer mind is full of waves like desires but our inner mind is calm and quiet. So the secret of peace is the knowledge of the self, and the thought "That this self only will help towards the gaining of a peace of mind which nothing can disturb.

The easiest meditation is transcendental meditation. This is simple because one doesnot have to control one's wandering mind by self-control. Here the thought is controlled by chanting of *mantras.* The most common mantra according to the Hindu religion is the *Gayatri Mantra.*

Gayatri is a Sanskrit word. Ga means to sing, Gyatri means protection. The word "Gayatri" has been defined as that which protects the vital air or life force or living force known as *pran.*

The omnipotent primordial energy (living force) is an independent creation of God. God has created the universe by dispersing energy throughout the universe. Hindus call this energy which is disbursed in the universe *Gayatri.* Thus *Gayatri* is the power of energy. The power which induces vibration, purifies thought-power, fills in us bubbling energy, which endows discrimination and sustains life.

The thoughts that arise in one's mind which are vicious and wandering constantly deplete the power of one's living force. It is like an engine that is always in use loses its energy and ultimately break down. The agitated mind weakens the mental power. Persons of a depleted living mental force do not really live in the true sense of good life.

To know the secret of the power of generating energy within us, we have to understand the tenets and disciplines of ancient

Indian Super *mantra*, which is nothing, but the twenty-four lettered "super-*mantra*, Gayatri. "Mantra" is a scientifically composed verse in the Sanskrit language, mostly composed of two lines with specific information for the invocation of divine powers.

Secondly, it is a combination of letters, which are sounds, or an arrangement of words with specific spiritual potentialities.

Mantra is vibration of spiritual words and when recited can pacify our minds.

Thirdly, these potentialities unfold themselves in the physical body as a result of the awakening of the power centers in the body which are called *chakras*.

This all happens because of the sound waves released by the repetition of the letters of the Mantra. Each time we recite the mantra the energy is released via sound waves. So the real power of the mantra lies hidden and is in the form of syllables, the uttering of the mantra repeatedly can awaken it.

Mantras contain powers and deep philosophical meaning and its singing repeatedly benefits mental, physical and spiritual health.

When we recite the Gayatri Mantra, we can feel it is endowed with extra-sensory, spiritual powers as well as mental powers. It has infinite power. It has a tradition and practice. It is the best medium for spiritual training. We get vital force in our body and new inspiration by reciting it.

The Science of Mantras

The whole mantra science is based on the combinations of sound waves and their frequencies. Each combination is in harmony with a particular power or power center within our body as well as with the subtle but very powerful energy center in the ethereal world. It is true that mantras are effective even when they are recited without being understood.

The simple explanation of this fact is that the meaning of mantras has an effect on thinking, and reciting subtle sound waves, which is a good tool of mental training. Moreover, various frequencies released by the utterance of the mantra have their effect on the potent power centers lying hidden in the spinal cords of the body. The reciter of the *mantra* is able to develop extra sensory powers simply by chanting the verse.

The science of sound holds that hidden in sound and what results from it can be achieved by its unknown vibrations. It is a proven fact that sound waves are like energy waves. These energies of *mantras* when channeled through our mind can fill our body with immense power which will cure all our diseases.

There are only three conditions, three stages, and three milestones to be fulfilled to materialize spiritual life, viz., *mantras.* They are: *Upasana* (true worship), *Sadhana* (correct life), and *Aradhana* (service to humanity). All three are inter-linked. You cannot have a correct life without worship and service to humanity. You cannot perform service to humanity without having compassion. Compassion can only be achieved via worship.

Upasana or Worship

The meaning of *upasana* is to close by. It is to sit close to God or the Inner Self. God is defined as Super Self within us. It is like two bodies within the same mind. One must change his life and surrender to the Inner Self. You will dance at the will of the inner self at this stage. If we achieve this stage we will have the advantage of becoming identical with God. Fuel is worth nothing, only when it embraces fire it becomes fire itself. We can achieve this stage by simply removing our ignorance of mind by light of *mantras*. When we feel separated from the world then we are in darkness and weak, but when we are united with every body via our inner self we are powerful and spiritual. It is just like kindling the fuel by our fire of our spirit.

Fire does not become fuel, fuel becomes fire. A drop of water merges into and becomes one with the ocean. The ocean does not become a drop.

Sadhana or Correcting Ourselves

Sadhana means taming or training of the mind. It can also mean conversion of a confused, scattered mind into a well-organized one. And it can also mean controlling of the senses and mind. It is also called the process of self-purification.

Greed leads one to cheat others. Temptation leads one out of control toward some desirous object. Ego illusion leads one to pride more than he has. Temptations of the tongue lead one to eat more and more of any unhealthy food. A man having these vices is bound to be dragged down. Man has five main senses—hearing, seeing, smelling, tasting and touching. Each sense is open outwards and each has its own vibration. If we always listen to their desires we are going to ruin ourselves.

One should maintain all-round self-restraint and discipline to eradicate these evil thoughts. Evil thoughts should be neutralized by good thoughts. Bad thoughts are mainly of habits and their usage while good thoughts always have the strong support of logic, facts, proof, wisdom, etc. Silencing of mind can cure worrying.

Aradhana or Service to Humanity

Aradhna means adoration. It pertains to devotion for the service of mankind. A person practising the principles of *aradhana* finds himself merged with every living being in the universe. Mahatma Gandhi was a great humanist as he did immense service for the uplifting of the poor and untouchables. Aradhana is the remedy for self centeredness which has created the most dangerous problems of the modern world.

We are unable to do service to the entire mankind due to limitations of time and money, but we can do the immense service to mankind by simply sending good thoughts to every one.

The most important lessons, which a soul has, learn living in this body are of *upasana*, *sadhana*, and *aradhana*. These paths lead man to the higher life.

The practitioner of Gayatri Mantra is blessed with all the qualities of the above elements.

The *mantra* that is to be chanted is "*Om Bhoor Bhuvaha Sawaha*" should be chanted silently for 10 to 15 minutes. Before practicing the *mantra* we should understand its meaning. *Om* is the symbol of God. When a man reaches a trance stage he will only hear the resounding of the word *Om*. It is the symbol of God according to Hindus whereas the words *Bhoor*, *Bhuvaha*, and *Swaha* represent creative, protective, and combative powers that are represented by "Bhoor", "Bhuvaha", and "Swaha" respectively. They also signify the three worlds, viz., the earth, the heaven, and the sub-terranean world. The entire universe is operating under three powers of God which are creation, protection and changing forms or death. Worshipping fire, air, and water and adopting the triple blessings of virility, dynamism, and peace within one's inner self, is where one's life can be made happy, prosperous, and peaceful in every way.

After chanting the mantra several times the three spiritual ideas of truth, love, and justice will emerge.

Tips for Preparing for Mantra Chanting

(a) Try to find 10 to 15 minutes of time away from your busy life.

(b) Sit quietly in a comfortable position. This means on a soft and hard surface.

(c) Set the clock for 15 minutes.

(d) Shut off the TV, radio, and telephone. Please tell your family members not to interfere in your chanting.

(e) Close your eyes.

(f) Relax your muscles.

(g) Focus on a mantra, if you want to chant your own religious mantra selects any mantra from your holy book (see below).

(h) Breathe slowly and naturally, when you inhale chant the mantra, when you exhale chant the mantra.

(i) When thoughts come to your mind, let that go with the chanting of the mantra. This will slow down the mind, and the mind will get energy.

(j) Practise this technique twice a day.

Judaism teaches chanting just like Hinduism does. Fourth and fifth century BC followers of a philosophy called Merkabolism would sit in a foetal-like posture and focus on breathing. They would repeat the same magic seal on each exhalation and disregard other thoughts when they came to mind.

In Christianity, repetitive prayers dating back almost to the time of Christ are evolved by word of mouth. These prayers are still practised in Byzantine monasteries.

Very similar practices are found within Islam, Buddhism, Shintoism, Taoism, Confucianism, with the only difference being in the words that are repeated. In Islam, the repetitive word of the Mantra is Allah, similar to the word Om. In Buddhism, the mantra of Gyatri is translated in the Lotus Sutra.

The Lotus Sutra version is "*Nam-myoho-renge-kyo*".

During the TM technique the mind settles down to a silent, yet fully awake state of awareness. At the same time, the body gains a unique and profound state of rest and relaxation.

This deep rest provided by TM eliminates the build-up of stress and tension, and provides the basis for more dynamic and rewarding activity.

The Maharishi comment: "In Transcendental Meditation, the conscious mind comes to a state of self-referral awareness, which is the simplest form of human awareness where consciousness is open only to itself. This self-referral state of consciousness is in the unified field of natural law."

When the conscious mind identifies itself with the unified field through the process of Transcendental Meditation, then human awareness is open to its own full potential, which is the total potential of nature's intelligence.

The practising of *mantras* allows the active thinking mind to settle down to transcendental consciousness, the field of pure intelligence, where the mind is silent, unbounded, and fully awake in itself.

The heart of Gayatri meditation is the sun. The Sun is the most powerful and dynamic planet in the solar system. Without the sun life cannot exist. According to psychology one who thinks and meditates on sun can become as powerful as the sun. When a person recites Gayatri Mantra, the sound waves travel inside the mind and vibrate the subtle part of the mind. This is a "Primordial energy" which can only be obtained by Gayatri chanting. It cannot be obtained by any physical science.

Dr Annie Beasant and Charles Leadbeater are leaders who did research on life after death and had the power to travel out of the body and also possessed power of seeing the invisible, unknown world with their naked eyes. They discovered that the flow of light from the sun of unseen matter goes towards the person reciting the Gayatri Mantra and makes him enlightened.

Brain Wave Coherence

One of the most significant findings pertaining to mantras has been the discovery that mantra chanting produces a unique ordering or coherence in brain wave patterns between the different parts of the brain.

Dr Wallace, who is a leading authority on this scientific research, explained the meaning of these findings.

He said that mantra chanting "optimizes brain functioning." This means that the brain functions in a more coherent, integrated style during chanting.

This higher EEG coherence gained is associated with increased intelligence, increased creativity, and higher moral reasoning.

The Gayatri Mantra does not belong to any particular sect of worship, nor is it restricted to any certain community. It is universal, for the whole world. It contains not only one culture but also cultures of the entire world and humanity. It is the treasure that belongs to the whole humanity.

We are living in an age of science. A modern mind is not easily prepared to accept anything as truth unless it is proved beyond doubt by scientifically approved methods. Science tries to explain the object by defining its characteristics, its structure, and its atomic structure. All these are defined by mind. If the mind is conditioned then the theory that is developed will not be really true; they are relatively true. Thus great scientists and philosophers of the present age have arrived at almost similar conclusions by scientific analysis that every object in the universe is the sum of its qualities and since qualities exist only in mind the whole objective universe of matter and energy does not exist except as a construction of consciousness.

Max Plank, the great physicist and discoverer of the Quantum Theory, lead to the conclusion "consciousness I regard is fundamental. I regard matter as a derivative of consciousness. We can't get behind consciousness. Everything we talk about, everything we regard to exist is consciousness." All the research of matter is done by mind where the consciousness exists. Without mind nothing can be done. Mind over matter has been an established fact.

Eddington, another great physicist and philosopher, also said that among the new properties with which we propose to experiment were the atom, which probably includes a rudimentary form of consciousness. The Mind of God in particular is to be regarded as infinitely extended throughout space and time.

The great scientists and philosophers of this century have arrived at almost similar conclusions by scientific analysis that every object in the universe is the sum of qualities and since qualities exist only in the mind, the whole objective universe of matter and energy does not exist except as a construction of consciousness, an edifice of the conventional symbols shaped by the senses of man.

What is Meditation

Meditation is adventure for peace, the greatest adventure the human mind can undertake in the path of tranquility. Meditation is just to be, not doing any action, no thought, no emotion. We just are and it is a sheer delight of peace and enjoyment. From where does this delight and peace come when you are not doing anything? We cannot see this delight anywhere but it is present at every place. It is uncaused, because existence is made of the stuff called joy. Meditation opens the door of the mind. It clears the clogging of ignorance around mind; when mind is open then infinite delight and peace will enter in our mind.

When we are not doing anything and all our thoughts are absent from our mind then we are in a state of meditation. Meditation is a state when all the thoughts are tamed and the person is in infinite happiness due to elimination of worries. When all our activities have ceased in our mind we are in a state of joy; and then in that state of joy we are doing our work; still we feel that we are not doing anything; then it is a true state of meditation. Once we have become aware of the way our being can remain undisturbed, then slowly we can do things keeping alert that our being is not stirred.

Meditation is not inaction. It is not that we have to escape from the world and the family. It simply teaches us a new way of life. Meditating mind is like an ocean where thoughts emerge like waves but die on the surface.

Our life actions are like a cyclone and we become a center of the cyclone. Like a wheel our life goes on and everyone of us is rotating like a wheel. So the cyclone of wheel of life goes on without disturbance; it goes on really more intensely with more joy, with more peace and calmness when we are just a watcher and not attached with any action simply seeing all that is happening around us. The wheel of life will run smoothly if we do not try to pull it in any direction by force of attachment.

When we think that we are not a doer of any action, but simply a watcher. This is the whole secret of meditation. Any action whether chopping woods, reading books, working in office, or running a factory, we are always in a state of meditation, when our mind is in peace and not attached with any actions. When we are centering we are not lost we are always in a state of meditation. In this world we cannot live without work, work without attachment is the meditation.

When we are watching something there are two things; subject and object. You cannot see a third witness who is your self, which is seeing both subject and object. When subject and object both merge in self then that is the true knowledge of the world. When we try to analyze object without merging with self then we cannot analyze it in true sense. That is why scientific research always changes with evolution of the mind.

The quality of observation, the quality of being aware and alert that is what meditation is. We cannot be alert if our mind is full with thoughts. In that case our observation will be distorted. When we are not aware, we are lost in wilderness and we do not know what is happening around us. So Meditation means awareness. Without awareness we cannot enjoy bliss.

Whatsoever we do with awareness is meditation. Action when it is performed with awareness always end up in success and people who are in the state of meditation while doing work are performing quality work.

The first step in awareness is that we should be very watchful of our body. Slowly one becomes alert about each gesture, each movement. And as we become aware about our body a miracle starts happening. Many tensions of our body, will disappear. Our body becomes more relaxed. Our body becomes more attuned. A deep peace starts prevailing and subtle energy will start flowing in the body. Our body has eight *chakras* situated in different systems and when we are aware of our body, energy will start flowing in all the *chakras* and we experience a serpent fire.

After awareness of our body then we should start becoming aware of our thoughts. The thoughts are subtler than the body. And when we become more aware of thoughts, then we will notice what is going on inside us. When we are aware of our thoughts then our thoughts instead of wandering like a bird will become like a timid animal.

We will find that thoughts are moving like clouds in the sky, and some thoughts like a black cloud eclipse the mind. We will see that our thoughts are in a state of turmoil. Our thoughts are jumping like a monkey. This causes lot of wastage of energy. As we are not aware, this whole madness goes on running like an under-current. It affects every action we are doing. And the sum total of it is going to be our life.

The very phenomenon of watching it changes the whole situation. Slowly and slowly the madness of thought will disappear. Chaos in the thoughts will form a certain pattern. It becomes more subtle and peaceful. And afterward deeper peace prevails. And when our body and mind are at peace we will see that we are attuned to each other. They are not running in different directions. We will see that mind and body are in accord. In this case mind and body are synchronized.

Physics also tells us the same thing that in the initial Big Bang. There was chaos of gases and they were in a state of great turmoil then the pattern started emerging and condensation of gases took place which resulted in the formation of stars. Patterns always develop after there is chaos.

When we are aware of our thoughts then there is one step more. A little more awareness is needed and we start reflecting our moods, our emotions and our feelings. Once we are aware of all these three they all become joined into one phenomenon. Unorganized thoughts are causing all the problems in us. When thoughts are under control then our emotions and moods are also under control.

Thoughts about our past, our present and future are causing that fear in us. When thoughts are streamlined and when we make them silent then we achieve a state of meditation.

And when all these three are one—function together perfectly—they are humming together. We can feel the music of all the three.

The important thing is that in meditation we are watchful, we are watching...watching...watching. And slowly, as the watcher becomes more and more solid, stable, unwavering, a transformation happens. The things that we were watching disappear.

Meditation originated from Yogis of India. It has now become a worldwide technique. We cannot learn it by force. It is growth of our total living. Meditation is not something that can be added to us as we are.

It cannot be added to us. It can only come to us through a basic transformation, a mutation. Meditation can be grasped by peaceful mind; it cannot enter in the mind where thoughts are in great stage of turmoil.

Meditation will bring a flowering a growth. Growth is always from the total; it is not an addition. Just like love, it can be added to us. It grows out of us, out of our totality. We must grow towards meditation. It grows from our silent mind and heart. It grows like a lotus flower, whose roots are on earth.

Lotus is not mingled with the mud of the soil. So is the meditation. It does not become affected with the dense thoughts.

Meditation is the silence of thoughts. People generally think that silence is negative, something empty, an absence of sound. Silence is positive. It is existential, it is not empty. Silence means that our mind will not allow entering of bad thoughts, the silent mind will burn down all the negative thoughts entering in our mind. Silent mind is overflowing with a music that we have never heard before. With a light that can only be seen by the inner eyes.

Our inner world has its own taste, its own fragrance, has its own light. It is utterly silent, externally silent. There has never been any noise. No word can reach there, but we can reach. It is like a black hole where anything entering in a black hole will disappear. Nothing can escape from it. People having that state of silence will experience timelessness. It is completely different than the outer world. The outer world is full of noise and turmoil and disturbance, whereas the inner world is silent and peaceful.

We are the very center of being. It is the center of cyclone. Whatever happens around it does not affect it. It is external silence. These internal silences always remain the same. It does not change due to change in time and space. It is like a middle and bottom of a sea where there is silence. There are no waves. They are only found on the surface of the sea.

Love, Meditation and Peace

If we meditate deeply, sooner or later we will feel a love. The emotion of love embraces us like a great force of attraction. Our heart will burn like a flame from which the radiation of love will move in all directions. Our heart becomes like a magnet where it will attract other loving hearts with great force.

If we love deeply then our circle of love starts increasing and expanding. By and by we will become aware that our love is becoming more and more meditative. We are going to be drowned in the ocean of love and subtle quality of silence is entering within us.

We find that our thoughts are disappearing, and we are touching our own depths. Love makes you meditative if it is on the right lines.

Today couples love each other for sex. Sex is called love. Soon the desire for sex fades away so does the love and they start fighting and eventually file for divorce. The cause of the depletion of love arises from lower mind. And lower mind will not give you glimpse of the external. Similarly, people have desire and love for money. Their desire burns like a fire and they are never satisfied. People will never find peace when they run for money and women.

Strong desire for anything is not love. This type of love always brings down man from higher level to the lower level.

First go on meditation and love will come out of meditation. Love that comes out of meditation is pure love. It is not sexual or money love. It is like a fragrance of flower coming out from meditation. Meditation is like a lotus flower with thousand petals, when it opens its fragrance will radiate in all directions. It is not directed to any one particular point. This fragrance of love will enter every place in the path of radiation. It will not discriminate anyone.

It is like the sunrays that will fall on every body who is in the path of that ray. Sunrays never discriminates anyone.

This is external love; it is unconditional. It is not a relationship; it is more quality that surrounds us. This is external love. It has been around Buddha, around Jesus, around Gandhi, around Krishna.

Compassion and Sympathy

Buddha said that compassion plays an important role in development of love. Compassion, according to him, equals love and meditation combined. He defined compassion as "love plus meditation". When love becomes selfless and when your love is sharing, and it is not asking any thing in return then this love becomes like an emperor mercy which spreads to every person without hoping for return.

When love is mixed with meditation then it is converted

into compassion. Sex is animal instruct whereas love is human and compassion is divine. Sex is physical, love is psychological, and compassion is spiritual. Mahatma Gandhi had a compassion for the untouchables of India. His meditation was uplifting the conditions of poor. This he achieved through the spirit of love for poor. His love was pure and divine due to which he was able to pinpoint his actions on uplifting of down-trodden people.

Intelligence

People who practise meditation will become intelligent and they will rediscover intelligence by following the path of meditation. The only method to rediscover it is meditation. Meditation eliminates all the barriers and images of the mind. When all the images and barriers are destroyed you will see the pure burning of a lamp of intelligence. Mind that is moving all the time with thoughts will loose all the power of intelligence and become dull. Take another example, water flowing on a wide range has weak flow but the same water is allowed to flow in a narrow pipe its flow becomes powerful.

Meditation simply removes all the blocks and saves us from being conditioned humous. It removes the rocks that are preventing our waters from flowing, our springs from becoming alive. Meditation is like a powerful spiritual wind, which blows out all the particles of resistance of our mind.

Meditation will pull us out from the cell of ignorance and will fill our mind with intelligence and love. Intelligence can be discovered through meditation.

When all these walls of ignorance cannot pollute our mind, when all these coverings of mind are removed, we become intelligent. After having undone what the society has done to us, we have become free humans.

Real Self

Meditation is also a device to make us aware of the real self which is hidden behind our layers of ignorance. When darkness of ignorance are removed by the light of meditation then real self will slowly emerge from behind and all the darkness of ignorance will be gone and the real self will shine. We are living with the unreal self, that is, our physical body which is going to die at the time of death. Real self, which is watching all the events, does not die after death. This real self is not changed due to change of space and time. It is a changeless self; we can experience it by means of meditation.

We will experience a unity of life. Meditation helps us to grow our own intuitive faculty. It becomes very clear what is going to fulfil us. The word 'personality' has to be understood. It comes from the root persona—persona means a mask. This is false mask when we do meditation this mask is removed.

The Three Essentials for Meditation

The three essential foe meditations are:

(1) Relaxed state, no fight with the mind; (2) Just watch the relaxed awareness whatever is going on; and (3) Watching the mind without any judgement.

These are the three things: relaxation, watching, no judgement. Then slowly and slowly a great silence descends over you. All movements are ceased.

Meditation is designed to relax the muscles of the body and to reduce the tension and anxiety within the body. It should never be done after heavy meal. In this case the inner energies (*pranic* energy) are busy in digesting the food. It will be difficult to channel it for meditation. Best time for meditation is morning. Allow your body to settle and you may prefer chair, bed or floor. Now, begin to notice your whole body and start thinking about it in a peaceful way. You will find that some of the areas of the body are tight and some are relaxed. Now, try to notice your breathing pattern. In this meditation of awareness exercise, take a deep breath with one nose closed and release it with another nose. Next, focus awareness of your feet. How they feel? Take a deep breath thinking about your toes, tighten the toes with inhale of breathing and release them while exhaling. Do this for three to five times.

Now, move your awareness to calves; then to your thighs. While gaining awareness of these body parts, try to make it tense with inhale breathing and release it while exhaling. This should also be done several times. Now, move your awareness to your stomach and intestinal region. Many times there is an anxiety stored in this part of the body due to which muscles of these parts contract. Consciously, relax your stomach and intestines by taking deep breath in and out. Feel your lungs expand and chest open as you breathe in and out. Try to do the same thing for your head. Head is the most complicated part of the body. In our head, the brain is running like a computer. Relax the brain by breathing in and out.

If your body is relaxed deeply because of these breathing exercises you will feel that a circle of healing light is surrounding you. Feel your body absorb the light. Take a moment to feel the peace within your body and your connection to this delightful light. Take one more deep breath before you end the meditation.

Do Your Work But Don't Look for Results

People have the ego and all the egos are result-oriented. I will work hard to get good raise or promotion. I will invest in stocks if I earn greater return.

People want to take action if there is positive outcome. People who are result-oriented often lose their mind if they don't succeed. Meditation happens only to those who are not result-oriented. Meditation is a non-goal-oriented state. Meditative people are steady in both success and failure.

While aware enjoy awareness and while unaware enjoy unawareness. Unawareness is like a rest. Unawareness means not thinking anything. It is a stage which is difficult to obtain. When you are unaware you are restoring the energy of the mind.

It is simple. Through unawareness awareness will rise again, fresh, young and this will go on. If you enjoy both you become meditative. You are not aware; not unaware but you are an enjoyer of both. In fact this is real enjoy. You are both enjoyer of sadness and happiness.

The same teaching Krishna gave in *Gita*. He said that a person who is unaware in both happiness and sadness is a real person who is dearer to God.

If happiness comes enjoy it, when sadness comes enjoy that too. How can you enjoy sadness? You can enjoy sadness if you think that the world of happiness and sadness are unreal as they are short lived and only real in this world is inner self which is not changing and unmoveable. If we enjoy sadness that sadness will be no longer sadness. It has become a silent peaceful moment, beautiful in itself. Later on you will find that we are enjoying neither happiness nor sadness. We are a watcher of every event. All the thoughts of darkness will be gone and it will not make us dirty as we are only a watcher of all events.

Appreciate Unawareness or Peace of Mind

Krishna said in *Gita* that a person who is not disturbed by pain and pleasure is a real person. A mind is like a powerful storm, which can blow all the peace and happiness of the man. Krishna said that curb the powerful mind by means of Yoga, or meditation. Person who has control of mind can experience doing nothing while actually they are doing their work.

Similarly, they who are not doing anything will feel they are doing something. In other words, while aware enjoy being aware and while unaware enjoy unawareness.

In meditation, a cycle of awareness and unawareness will follow. When you are meditating you will feel unawareness then after a while awareness comes, then when waves of awareness fizzle out then unawareness comes with full force. If you can enjoy both then your mind is in perfect state of equibrilum.

A person whose mind is not disturbed in happiness or sadness is the real person. The state of sadness and happiness are like heat and cold, which come and go and real persons are not disturbed by the waves of sadness and happiness. Then you find the ultimate reality where you will not find both happiness or sadness but you are separate from them and you are watcher of happiness or sadness.

Once this point is reached you are not crying when sadness comes and you are not celebrating when happiness falls. At this point you are celebrating life and death at the same level.

According to J. Krishnamurti in the whole life when the observer becomes the observed, know that you have arrived. Before that there are thousands of things on the way. The body gives its own experiences, which have become known as the experiences of the centers of *kundalini*. Seven centers become seven lotus flowers. Each is bigger than the other and higher, and the fragrance is intoxicating. The mind gives you great spaces, unlimited, infinite. But remember the fundamental maxim that 'still the home has not come.'

Enlightenment is not an experience. It is the state where you are left absolutely alone with complete silence. Only in that moment does your consciousness, unobstructed by any object, takes a turn and moves back to source.

This state of Nirvana is attained by deep meditation. In this state you will feel the unity of all lives. Buddha attained this state of mind by deep meditation. When the observer is the observed, when the knower is the known, when the seer is the seen, then home has arrived.

7

Meditation Through Brow *Chakra*

This *chakra* is situated above the eyebrows, in the center of the forehead. It affects the pituitary gland, the brain, the nervous system, and hormone-balance.

It is the center of insight and understanding, clairvoyance, awareness of spiritual potential, true creativity in the spiritual realm.

This is also called the third eye of a man. Between the two eyes there is a third eye existing, but ordinarily it is non-functional. You can open this eye by practising meditation.

Sit down on a mat on the floor. Unplug all telephones for 20 minutes. Now, close your eyes, and then focus both your eyes just in the middle of both eyes. Thinking that white light or powerful energy is focused on the third eye, that is focus on the middle of both eyes.

This is one of the simplest methods of being attentive. If you practise this technique you become hypnotized with the third eye.

This third eye catches attention. It is like a magnet, and when magnet is magnetized it attracts opposite polarity. So this third eye will be magnetically drawn, attracted, pulled by the gland itself.

So just close your eyes. Let your two eyes move just in the middle, and feel the point. When you are near the point, suddenly your eyes will become fixed. If you have a problem in locating the third eye then you should sit near a big mirror; after sitting in a comfortable pose then look through the mirror on the center of the two eyes. Concentrate on the center for few minutes, then close your eyes while you are still visualizing the center. For the third eye you will feel thoughts running before you; you will become witness. It is just like a film screen. Once your attention is focused at the third eye center, you are witness of a flowing thought. Since you have concentrated your mind on third eye the flowing thoughts are not going to bother you.

Ordinarily, if you are not a witness or you have not silenced your mind then you are flowing with thoughts and you are a thought, if angry thought flows then you are angry. If you are not a witness you become a part of a thought, and you take the form of thought. When sex is there you want sex, when greed thought is there you become greedy. You do not have any gap between you and the thought. Like water in the clouds is not separated the clouds look dark but when water is separated from the clouds then clouds disappear and sun comes out. Similarly, when thoughts are separated from our mind then light of real self will shine.

When you focus on the third eye you are separated from the thought, thought is running behind you, you are the witness. By separating your self from thoughts you are safe from loosing energy. You will gain lot of energy. When you are using the essence of breathing, you are not only breathing air. Science says you are only breathing air—oxygen, hydrogen, and other gases in the combined form of air. The air that we breath is the source of our life. It pumps the life energy in our body and soul due to which we survive. The air also contains force call "*Prana*" which is called life energy.

Hindu Vedas say that air is just a vehicle, not the real thing. Vedas say that you are breathing *Prana* not air. By simply focusing on the third eye you are observing the *prana*. When you are on the point when you observe "*PRANA*" you will experience lightness and become energized. After long practice you can be able to open your third eye then you will be able to see the future. You can predict the happenings of future. You can see even in darkness, and you don't need light to see the object. Your spiritual potential will rise.

Meditation for Rising Energy to Head

In this method rising energy from the spine or the sex center is done by methods of meditation. In the body the spine is a very important part. Its lower end is at sex center and the upper end is at the crown *chakra*.

This spine is a very important part of the body. If the spine is strong you have a strong mind and body. If it is weak then you are dull and inactive.

This spine connect the sex center to the crown *chakra*. These are two opposite polarities. Sex organ is connected with the earth, the material, whereas crown *chakra* is divine it is inactive for ordinary people. These two poles will determine the faith of your life.

Since the sex organ is very strong and its attraction is downwards; your life will be sex-oriented or divine-oriented. This sex energy is a strong force for all the creatures. This sexual energy is creative energy if it is channeled properly. Generally, when someone is engulfed with sexual desires he discharges his energy by performing sex. This sexual act is the wastage of energy. Yogis in India by means of yoga channeled the sexual energy to the mind. In upward journey to the mind the sexual energy passes through all the centers of *chakras* in the body and made them activated. Either your energy will be flowing down from the sex center or it is moving upwards and when it reaches the crown *chakra* then this energy will be released from the crown *chakra* outward into absolute existence.

When your energy moves downwards then you are loosing energy whereas if your energy moves upwards you will glimpse happiness and bliss.

When your energy is on its upward journey and it reaches at the crown *chakra,* it will experience the enjoyment of absolute bliss. So the whole effort of Yoga is to move the energy upward through the vertebrae, through the spinal column, this movement be against the gravity. Sex is very easy because it follows gravitation. The earth is pulling everything down. Your sex energy is pulled by earth.

You must have heard that astronauts when they cross the

axis of gravity their sexuality dissolves, disappears. When one of the astronauts when crossed the earth gravitation, he felt immense happiness. He saw earth as green with full of shining light. All the boundaries of countries disappeared.

The earth is pulling your life energy down and this is natural, because the life energy comes from the earth. All food you eat comes from earth. All these energies are pulled by earth. Everything is going on source. And if it continues to move in this way, life energy going back again and again, you are moving in a circle; you will go on moving for lives and lives. You can go on moving this way infinitely unless you take a jump just like astronauts.

Like the astronauts you have to take a jump then the circle of earth gravitation will be broken.

The techniques for how it can be broken are successful when the energy can move vertically and rise up within you, reaching new centers.

When this light reaches on the top at crown *chakra* we are completely changed people. We become divine like Buddha, Krishna and Gandhi. All the bodies of those great people broke the gravitation pattern of the earth. How to break this pattern of sexual life towards divinity is the lesson of this chapter.

In order to understand the sexual activity we find that sexual impulse will not arise without thinking. Sex energy moves with imagination. Just through imagination sex energy started moving up.

Imagination is very important for moving sex energy from one point to another. You cannot move your blood by imagination, but you can get ejaculations through imagination of sex. So sex energy can move so that we can change its direction.

As mentioned earlier we have seven centers. First is root *chakra*, which is related with sex. Seventh center is crown *chakra* and there are five centers within it. The second center is situated behind the navel, the third center upward from navel and below heart, fourth is on center of the heart, fifth is called the throat *chakra* which is in the throat, sixth is called the Brow *chakra* which is also called the third eye, the seventh is called Crown *chakra* which is on the head.

Imagine first that rays of light are entering through your body and it is rising from the sex center. As science said that everything is light, all elements are active due to electron and protons revolving round the nucleolus. Concentrate on your sex center that light is rising from this center. Now imagine that this light rays are moving up from the sex center to the navel center. From this navel center the rays are moving up towards the heart center, then towards brow and then towards head.

As the lights are moving from the sex center towards navel like the flow of river of light water. You will notice that after concentration at that point your navel center will become hot. You can feel the hotness. Now the light moves from the navel center to heart center, you will notice your life beat will increase, your flow of love will spread like a wild fire. Heart is the center of love. Now from the warmth of the heart it will rise to throat-you will experience inspiration and telepathy, then you will raise the level of light to eyebrows you will experience awareness of spiritual potential. Then when it reaches the head you will experience true cosmic awareness.

You must be wondering how these things are happening. Sex energy has two parts—one is physical and another is psychic. Physical part is semen, which cannot rise, and there is also the psychic part which controls the flow of semen.

This psychic part rises from the sex center and moves up the ladder. That psychic part uses the spinal passage to reach different centers. Sexual energy is activated by thought. Imagine your first sex intercoursed then your entire body will be filled with sexual energy.

The sexual energy is generated from the root *chakra* and then it is elevated to higher centers by force of meditation and finally it reaches the crown *chakra* where it dissipates outside by revolving spokes of crown chakra. The crown *chakra* has 296 spokes. When this energy reaches on the crown center its 296 revolving spokes spread the energy at every place.

This ascending energy will create sensitivity and feeling. You will also experience love instinct arising from you. This energy, when it arises from the root *chakra* should not be blocked by any center. Any blockage of rising energy will reduce the voltage of energy and will reduce its momentum. So in order to eliminate the blockage you should sit in a peaceful place. There should not be any disturbance in the near meditation place. In order to enjoy the full benefit bring this energy to your head and you will feel that the head has an opening.

In India and in ancient Vedas the crown *chakra* is compared with thousand of lotus petals. Since lotus is grown in mud and rises from the mud and receives an energy from the sunrays and then blooms, lotus petals are unaffected by any mud from the ground. Similarly, crown *chakra* arises from the head; Our body is full of passion, hunger, and sexual desires. So a person who is unaffected by these is like a lotus flower which is not affected by mud. Imagine that you are like a lotus and thousands of petals are emerging from your crown *chakra*. All these light energies you are receiving from the sex *chakra* or root *chakra* are thrown in to cosmos by the thousand petals of the *chakra*.

There are two types of orgasms. One is sexual and another is spiritual. Sex energy when not elevated is just a lower energy, but when it is moved up it becomes a spiritual energy. But do not leave the energy somewhere in the body at some center. When you are doing this meditation do not let any one to disturb you. Hook off the telephone and put the signboard "Please don't disturb". If you leave the energy somewhere in the ascending *chakra* it will cause harm in the mental set-up. The energy must come to the head, and should be released from there.

When you start meditation first you will feel much sexual impulse which will have powerful impact on your mind. But as the meditation becomes deeper, you will feel the energy flowing up. As the energy flows, the sex center becomes silent and less excited.

When this energy reaches at the peak of the head then there will be no sensation at the sex center. Sensation of the sex center is moved to the head. Sex center will become silent.

The hotness of the sex center has moved to the head but here it is not so hot. Due to meditation hotness has evaporated and converted into spiritual energy due to interactions with so many centers. Sometime this will cause your head to become little hot and cause some dizziness. You will also feel sleepy due to this. After that sleep you will feel so fresh that it is as if you have been a sleep for the first time, in the deepest slumber.

This is called Yogic sleep. It is a very deep sleep as you had moved to the deepest center. This caused you to feel as if your head is opening like a lotus flower, as if energy is being released into the cosmos. As the energy is released, it will bring coldness coming to our head. You have never felt the coldness that comes after this hotness. But do the technique completely; never do it incompletely.

So feel that energy; you will feel warmth as well as lovingness. A new life is coming to you, an inward light rising up. You will feel the light and you will feel peace of mind. Our mind will be full of power. It can do much wonderful mental work, which could not be done before. Only feeling backed by imagination will give good result.

Finding Inner Peace

Man's mind is always full of desires. Desires are roaming like clouds in a sky. As clouds cover the shining sun, so do the desires and unending thoughts cover the powerful mind.

The thoughts will pull you back into the past where you will be disturbed by some unpleasant incident. Then your desire or thoughts will push you into the future where you will fall in trap of illusory imagination. You will build up big plans of enjoyment and never be in the present moment of making it successful. Desire is always the cause of disturbance. It is like a disease. Peace comes when the mind is undisturbed. When you stop thinking about past and do not fall in the future thinking and always be in present moment then you have reached the stage of timelessness.

How to stay undisturbed in grip of violent disturbance is very important in your life. When you are angry you are in grip of anger. You are mad, you start planning to take revenge and you are disturbed.

Suddenly remember to be undisturbed—you have to get rid of anger then you will be peaceful. Your anger is wavering on the periphery of your mind. It is rising and falling on the outer surface of the mind. It is like sea waves, which rise and fall on the seashore but middle of the sea is calm and quiet whereas the higher mind is undisturbed. Just like sea waves, which appear only near the shore, but if you go inside the sea you will find no waves. There will be still waters and entire sea will be calm like an unwavering air.

Let the anger rise and fall at the periphery and let your higher mind be the witness of your anger. As you reach the center of your mind you will find peace.

When you feel angry you have two options. Firstly, you may focus your thought on an object that causes anger. Your vibration of anger focus may shift on an another person, which stirred your peace and due to which you are angry. Imagine that the other man is also angry with you, he is also harbouring angry thoughts on you. So your mind which is in grip of anger will suddenly receive another wave of anger vibrations that will have a cumulative effect on your mind and you will become more mad.

Secondly, instead of moving your anger outside let your thought travel inside. Instead of moving on the object let it move on the subject, that is yourself. If you move to the object, the dust part of the mind is disturbed and you will feel disturbed and in conflict with self. If your thoughts travel within yourself you will notice that you are the witness of your anger and you will find that your outer mind is disturbed but inner mind is calm and quiet. When these outer layers of anger will disappear then you will see the shining inner mind. It does not mean that you are storing the anger within yourself. You are only dissolving that anger in the calmness and peace of mind.

A sexual desire comes to your mind, your whole body start shaking. You move your sexual desires to your object of sex. You will find more disturbances. The further you go away from the center you will feel more disturbed. Really, the distance and disturbance are always in proportion. The more you are away from the center you are more disturbed. As you are nearer to the center you are less disturbed. If you are just on the center you are undisturbed and peaceful. Many people perform rape when they cannot curb the desire of sex.

In a cyclone, there is a center which is undisturbed—similarly in the cyclone of anger and cyclone of sex, there is a center where there is no anger, and there is a point in a cyclone of sex where there is no sex.

Remember that God has created two opposites all the time. Without opposite there will be no life. The magnet has two polarities—positive and negative. At the center of a magnet there is no polarity. So there is a center within you which is calm and unmoved. There is an outer layer, which is in grip of intense disturbance. You have free choice either to adopt peace or adopt disturbance.

When you are in the grip of anger you have to be undisturbed. This does not mean that you have to suppress anger. Suppression will cause more harms. We are just separating our mind from the anger. Take for example, in white milk pour little oil; oil will not dissolve in the milk oil and milk will be separated on the surface. Similarly we have to separate anger from the mind.

We have to confine our anger on self and not let our anger move out. We have to dissolve the madness of anger in the cold and infinite peaceful mind. Just let the force of anger dissolve in the mind and then its energy will be peaceful. Take for example if we throw red colour in the moving water of river the red colour will dissolve in the water.

Meditate on the anger and think of some past incident of anger and how you had diffused it. When you diffused the anger then you remain undisturbed, rather than when you suppress it. Diffusing the anger is like releasing of vapour from the pressure-cooker.

Expression and suppression are easy; witnessing is difficult. Witnessing is neither suppression nor expression. Witnessing means we are looking on a flow of anger in our mind. It is not expressing because we are not expressing it to the object of anger. Expression will explode like a bomb and it is going to destroy us. It is not being suppressed either. We are allowing it to be expressed in a vacuum. We are meditating on it.

Suppose we are angry then we should go near the mirror and express our anger on ourself. Imagine this anger had arisen due to some of our mistake. We can let the wave of anger flow on us so that it is not allowed to move out. If we want to beat someone beat the empty drum. We can diffuse the anger by sending peaceful thoughts from some previous happenings.

If we want to scream we should scream alone. Reminding ourselves that this is drama. Our screaming on one will release the screaming energy. Our mind is a like an ocean in which all the rivers of screams and anger flow and dissolve in it.

By this practice we will notice that there is a center or point which is undisturbed. Now, try to uncover this center more and more.

Take a magnet, you will find two polarities at its end. One is positive, another is negative, but the center is neutral; it is neither positive nor negative. So there is center in us where two forces working simultaneously give us transcendence, and then in real anger also we cannot feel it. This is the real test. In any world situation if the anger comes we remain undisturbed.

So, when we are at the center then this will give us energy and happiness. Then nothing can create any confusion in us, nothing can hurt us. Once we detach our center from the outer layer of anger, then anger will not disturb us.

This technique is to experience two extremes within our self. When we realize that there are two extremes in our body then we will become a master of ourself.

If we do not practise it we will be slaves of the situation. If we can be happy and unhappy because of someone else then we are slaves of those people. If we are not disturbed by pulling of strings by others then we are real masters of ourselves. If somebody by simple gesture, can make us unhappy. Just by a simple smile he can make us happy. So we are just at the mercy of someone else. Then we are slaves of so many people. Any one can pull us down. If we are not disturbed by somebody's action then we are free and not slaves.

Revive Energy by Neutralizing Sound Waves

We are living in a world of sounds. At every place honking of a car, television noise, the loud noise of flying planes, even the vibration of vacuum cleaner all are disturbing us in our day to day life. Many people do not want to lung a house near the airport due to adverse noise. Generally, sound waves moves in a circle, they do not travel in a straight line. All sounds move in a circular path. All circles have a center.

Imagine that we are the center of all the sound waves. The sound is moving towards us in a circle. We are taking bath of sounds at the center. Feel as if every sound is moving towards us and we are the center. This imagination that we are the center of all the sound waves will give us deep peace. The whole universe becomes the circumference and we are the center of every thing. At the center the sound waves will not disturb us. It can only disturb us when we are away from the center.

If we are sitting near a waterfall, we will hear the sounds of water. Imagine that those sounds are entering in our ear from all sides. It is moving in a circular wave. The greatest advantage of being the center of a circle is that we become soundless. A sound cannot hear another sound. Since we become a center of a sound so we cannot hear any sound.

This center is absolute silence: that is why we can hear sounds, entering us, coming to us, penetrating in us, encircling us. Since we are center of a sound we are not hearing any sound.

First, you have to find out where the center is? Then at that point you will find all the sound is disappearing. That is the point you will feel soundlessness. This is the center of life. When we reach a center then we are deaf to the outside world. Then we can hear the sounds of our heart.

Once we are at the center, then no sound can disturb us. Sound waves come near us but are never able to disturb us. There is a point where no sound enters. That is our point. When we reach that point we will gain lot of energy. Sounds of different types cannot disturb our concentration.

When we find the point of silence we will experience waves of energy emerging from our center. That energy can open our *chakras* and we will float in waves of energy that will emerge within us.

Sounds are not heard in ears. Ears are just a transmittal of sound. And in this transmission they select only certain sounds, which fall in certain frequencies. The center of a sound is in the brain. The center of a brain where sound waves become silent is found with practice of yoga and meditation.

For instance in a temple, a man is meditating, many people come and ring the bell and the sounds are created and these sound waves enter the ears of the meditator. This does not disturb the meditator. The sound waves enter at the center and disappear. The disappearing sound waves left silent energy, which help the meditator to fall in deep meditation.

If sound is the vehicle to move to the other, then soundlessness becomes the vehicle to move to oneself.

With sound you communicate with others, with soundlessness you fall down to our own abyss. Try to understand these sound waves then we will find that soundlessness will move within.

Concentration

Concentration is another method of calming the mind and feeding energy into it. In concentration the mind is focused on one object. It is another form of meditation in which the mind can become powerful by one pointed concentration.

The mind is run by thoughts. All these thoughts run outward. Thought jumps from one object to another. Such monkey mind needs to be controlled. While the mind is collecting material for thought, many people think that the mind cannot live without mobility, and they think that it is difficult to curb the mind, it just likes controlling the strong flowing wind.

They think that the stoppage of this mobility by means of concentration on a single object seems impossible. The mind which receives images of outer objects through the brain is busy in interpretation and doing modifications of the objects depending on the conditioning of our brains. We cannot see the true image due to conditions of the mind. Take for example, if you see the world with a red glass everything will look red, whereas every object is not red. The wandering mind loses all energies and becomes weak. Take for example, if the battery is used all the time it will loose its power and need recharging.

In concentration, consciousness is held at one point or on a single image. In this case, the entire concentration of the mind is fixed on one single object, the wavering mind only wavers on a single object now. The mind which runs and is attracted by external object jumps from one object to another, now stands alone on a single object, disregarding all the impressions thrown upon it. It is just like chaining a dog at one place.

Now, when mind is kept shaped to one image, and the individual understands it, he understands it better than any reading or verbal description of the object. Constant observation of any object will unlock the mystery of that object and you can grasp the object easily.

Words are symbols of things; words describe the object from outside whereas concentration grasps the object more deeply, where words cannot enter. It must be remembered that concentration is not a state of passivity, but on the contrary one of regulated and intense activity. By means of concentration one can penetrate inside the object and glimpse the inner structure of the object. Many scientists were able to find the new theories by means of concentration on that subject.

At the beginning of concentration two difficulties arise. First, the mind is wavering and starts answering the image of different thoughts. In this case the mind is detracted by many different thoughts. The thoughts are deflected from the object on which we want to concentrate. So when thoughts are wandering and deflecting from the object then it is wasting lot of energy. Therefore the mind should be stopped from deflecting from the object and it should be arrested inside and resisted to outside image. The mind should stop responding to outside images. But stopping the reply of images sometimes causes resistance in the mind. We must balance and be in a perfect state of equilibrium between two resistance and non-resistance forces.

We should make our mind still and be steady. The quietitude should be so strong that waves from outside will not produce any result, not even a slight vibration.

Secondly, the mind itself holds the sole image, for the time, the object of concentration. We should not let outer thoughts modify and condition the object which we are concentrating. It must not only refuse to modify itself in response to impacts from outside. If it is allowed wandering then it will cease its inner activity and power.

The mind is now confined to its attention to a single object, to fix itself there. The mind focuses all its activity on a single object then it gets the power. Take for example, the water flowing over a wide surface has little impact on a motor power but the same water sent along a narrow channel, with same initial impulse, will carry away an object. Similarly, steam allowed to expand in free air does not move any thing, but if the steam is allowed to pass through a pipe, the same steam runs a piston with great force.

Hence, the value of concentration is continually insisted on by the yogis and teachers of meditation. It greatly enhances strength of the mind. If the mind is wandering, it wastes lot of mental energy, but if the mind is allowed to concentrate then it gains energy and does miracles. Turning the mind outside is easy, our mind is attracted towards many external objects, but allowing the mind to enter inside is not an easy thing. All our nine gates of senses open outside and all of them are controlled by brain, which always throw the sensations outside and brain is controlled by lower mind.

This lower mind also enjoys outer physical vibrations.

In our inner compartment we have a self who is a ruler and our mind is slave. In most of cases this slave rules the master, and we become a helpless victim of passions.

How Consciousness Works in our Body

In the object world every object occupies certain space and

has a position which depends on X and Y coordinates. A body can be moved, then it occupies another space. This transition may be swift or slow or medium speed. Every physical object has limitation of space and time. This limitation of space and time limits our ability in our performance and our freedom.

Now, regarding consciousness there is no limitation of space. It travels from one place to another in flash of a light. A solid body has a limitation of space and weight. One body only attracts another body depending upon the distance. If the distance is increased then attraction between the objects is decreased. Attraction is inversely proportional to distance.

In case of consciousness there is no such limitation of space. It can go from one place to another within a fraction of a second.

A person can concentrate on any object even on the other planet, not because his astral vision acts telescopically, but because in the inner region the whole universe exists as a point.

Such a man reaches the heart of life, and sees all things therein.

It is written in a Hindu *Upanishad* that within a chamber of heart there is a small chamber, and in it there exists a self which is immortal and the same cosmic energy of self existed all over the universe, including sky, sun, moon, galaxies, fire, stars, etc. Emission of heat by sun, the rotations of planets around the sun, movement of galaxies are all controlled by the same super energy which existed in our body as silent and inactive force which is called self. The *Upanishads* state that the entire universe is running with the power of self, which is also present in our heart.

So this self which is truly one and all pervading, so that anyone who is conscious in the self is conscious of all points of the universe? Physics stated that a movement of a body will affect the farthest star, because all bodies are inter-connected by ether which is a continuous medium which transmits vibration without friction or without any loss of energy. Any vibrations generated in a body are transmitted to other bodies depending upon how powerful the vibrations are. Generally, the vibration will die out as distance is travelled.

This is one form or physical side of a story. How natural, then, it is that consciousness which is the life side of nature, should be similarly all pervading and continuous. We feel ourselves to be here, other objects of the universe influence us. If our consciousness is fully developed then we can influence any far object of universe in a way as any object inside the room.

Concentration is the means whereby the soul escapes from bondage of forms and enters in peace. "For him, without concentration there is no peace."

The light of self shines through all, provided we generate power within ourselves to grasp the shining lights of others. We can enjoy warmth of spiritual energy which is much more powerful than any wilderness of forms.

Man is the creation of thought; what he thinks upon in this life, that hereafter, he becomes. Thought is the building block of any design of object. Take for example an engineers thinks a design of building in the mind first then he gives concrete form of that building. Physical body that we have got is the result of our past *karma* of previous life.

How to Concentrate?

At a clean spot, which is neither too high nor too low, a seat should be made with tight cloth and soft pillow.

Firmly seated on it, the Yogi should practise spiritual communion, with inner self and mind should be concentrated with the help of working of the imaginative faculty and senses should be under control for self-purification. The senses will try to detract the mind. In that case a Yogi or the person should try to concentrate again in the inner self.

Holding the body, head and neck erect, motionless and firm, gazing at the tip of the nose and round-about, fearless, serene, restrained in mind, and established in the vow of continence, he should sit in spiritual communion with inner self.

With the mind restrained from going outward to objects and always uniting with the inner self, the Yogi attains to Peace, which is the summit of bliss.

This concentration or Yoga is not for those who eat too much, nor for those who eat too little. It is neither also for those given too much sleeping, nor for those who keep too much vigil. For one who is temperate in food and recreation, who is detached and self-restrained in work, who is regulated in sleep, these type of people can easily practice Yoga.

When the disciplined mind is able to remain established in the Self alone, when it is free from longing for all objects of desire- then it is spoken of having attained to spiritual communion. The flame of a lamp sheltered from wind does not flicker. This is the comparison used to describe a Yogi's mind that is well under control and united with Self.

This state in which mind with its movements restrained by the practice of concentration, finds rest in which a person experienced the joy of the spirit born of the higher mind and communicating with the Self. A person who practices concentration should abandon imagination-born longings in their entirety, restraining all the senses with the mind on every side, and setting that mind firmly on the Self alone. One should then find the tranquillity in that state when his mind is absolved from every kind of thought.

No doubt, the mind is fickle, turbulent, powerful and unyielding like a storm. To control it is as difficult as controlling the powerful wind. Undoubtedly, the mind is fickle, and wandering like a cloud this makes it difficult to check. Yet, it can be brought under control by dispassion and spiritual practice.

The Yoga is difficult of attainment by men of uncontrolled mind. But for those who have their minds under control, they can master the techniques of Yoga and it is possible to attain perfect Nirvana, if they strive with proper means.

Yoga asserts unity of all existence at the level of higher Self in a planet of all lives and defines Spiritual Self and emphasizes the intimate relation between that Spiritual Self and individual Self.

Self-centeredness and ego go away when one finds the same Self in all. One will experience pain by seeing the suffering of other people and feel joy when he sees the joy of others. Psychologically it shows that spiritual intuition, which Yoga gives, enables man to increase his sphere of influence and has a distinct content of unique nature and is not mere fantasy without any life-enhancing value.

There are two aspects to the Self of a man—the higher and lower. The higher Self is called higher mind turned towards the Self whereas the lower self is the mind dominated by the senses. It is said the sense-dominated mind should not be allowed to overcome the higher mind. The higher mind should draw strength from the Self by communion with it. When the higher Self controls the senses then we are the master of the game. According to Krishna our work will be successful and bad cause and effect do not limit us. Our higher Self always shows the correct path.

Mindfulness

Mindfulness is the other major classification of meditation practice, known as *Vipassana*, or insight meditation. In mindfulness a person starts a meditation by utilizing one-pointed attention to cultivate calmness and stability. When thoughts and feelings come up a person should not suppress the thought, but observe the thought as it passes. Just observe the thought without any judgement and intention. In this meditation thoughts are not allowed to suppress, as the founder of this technique believes that suppressing the thoughts will generate more resistance in the mind and should not be encouraged. Thoughts should not be allowed to be suppressed. They should be observed as they pass the brain. You will find that these thoughts are roaming in the brain like clouds in a sky. When bad thoughts and depression cloud our brain we should immediately replace them with good thoughts. This will give soothing vibration and peace of mind. Slowly, we can get rid of all thoughts.

Paradoxically, this inclusive nothing of thoughts that come and go in our mind can lead us to feel less caught up in them and give us a deeper perspective on our reactions to everyday stress and pressures. Actually, thoughts are the reflection of our daily stress and emotions.

We should not be drowned in the deep depression of thoughts. Thought, if they strikes our mind should be allowed to move in the mind and we should be the silent watcher of that movement. If we are unable to be silent watcher then we should replace it with good thoughts.

By observing our thoughts and emotions we can observe how these thoughts are made up or how the emotions and attachments are flowing in the thought waves. The thoughts of people who are ego-centric are always self-centered and cover. the aura with depression and close our mind from outside subtle thoughts.

We also observe dislike, hatred and depressions which we experienced sometime in past. By watching these thoughts we can find out our own weakness of judgement in our actions. These thoughts are reflection of our world, which we see by our selfish mind. By analyzing these thoughts we can correct our past mistakes and prevent them from occurring in future.

The key to mindfulness is that we choose to focus on quality of awareness that we experience each moment. That awareness will vitalize our mind and give peace in the mind. It is very important that this awarenesses—will be non-judgmental—more of silent witnessing, a neutral observer, than running commentary on our inner experience.

Observing without judging, moment by moment, helps us in what we see on our mind without censoring it, without getting lost in our own incessant thinking. The goal of mindfulness is for us to see what is happening in our own body and mind at that particular moment. If we experience a distressing thought or feeling of actual physical pain at any moment by observing we can reduce the heat of the thought wave. The observance of thoughts will help us in reducing our tension. We can correct the distressed thoughts by good thoughts.

Acceptance of the roaming thoughts course does not mean passivity or resignation. On the contrary, by fully accepting what each moment offers, we can open ourselves to experiencing life much more completely and make it more likely that we will be able to respond effectively to any situation that presents itself. Responding to the current situation and being alert from moment to moment is important for success and peace of mind. If we don't observe our thoughts then we will never be able to know our weakness and strength of mind. When we know our weakness of mind then we can correct it and be able to be successful in our actions.

One way to envision how mindfulness works is to think of mind as the surface of a lake or ocean. There are always waves, sometimes big, sometimes small.

These waves in the surface of the lake do not disturb the calmness of water at the center of a lake. Similarly, do not let the waves of thought on the outer rim of the mind disturb the calmness of your inner mind. In some meditation it is advised to stop and check the rising of waves but in this technique of mindfulness waves are not allowed to stop but to learn a lesson from the rising waves by watching it inside a mind. Watching the waves of thoughts reflects our inner motion of weakness and strength.

There are two methods of practising this meditation. One is the formal method which involves specific techniques to help us keep our focus on the present moment in extended period of time. Focusing on the present moment eliminates all the worries of the past and makes it successful in our present efforts. Informal practice it is also simply reminding us to be in the present moment during daily activities. Informal practices only draw our attention to the present moment.

Formal Practices

This is similar to concentration described above. Like concentration we focus a series of focal points. Whatever the object of attention, it does not take long before the mind wanders off, even though we fully intended to keep it in one place. Each time it occurs before refocusing our attention. We must observe as non-judgmental as possible before mind went off and then gently bring our mind back to the object of our attention in the meditation. It is just playing hide and seek with the thoughts. Bring the mind back on the object of focus if it is carried away by thought. It is method of arresting a thought at a particular point. Thoughts are not allowed to wander from place to place. Constant focusing on certain point energizes our mind. It is like forcing a gas on a narrow chamber where all the gases like to exit at the same time from the hole, which result in higher speed and force. Same gases when roaming on a wider pipe have slows speed and force.

This resembles one-pointed meditation in that we are bringing our mind back to a particular focus. Whether it is the breath or something else, there is an important extra feature. We are nothing. By physical distraction we can bring our mind to particular point.

In this formal meditation body scan is done. We scan our attention through the various regions of our body. We can do this meditation as follows :

This is a good way of reviving our *chakras*. We usually begin by choosing a single object of focus—for example our breathing. We can concentrate on one aspect of our breathing, such as feeling of the air as it passes in and out of our nostrils or the gentle expanding and deflating of our body with each in-breath and out-breath.

Sit comfortably, with your back and neck straight, eyes closed, inhale a white sunlight through your right nose after shutting the left side of the nose, hold the breath and imagine that sunlight is on your base center, count up to 10, or if you don't want to count then hold the breath for 15 seconds and exhale the breath through your left nose after closing your right nose with count of 10 or exhale it in 15 seconds. Repeat this process three times. Each time we assume that our base center is illuminated by sunrays. This way we feel the glow of base center. This is the same way of energizing the *kundalini*.

Now, raise the consciousness to the spleen center, imagine again the white sun light is entering our body, inhale the breath with your left nose keeping you right nose closed, and assume the white ray of light is illuminating your base center. Hold the breath there for five seconds or count of four. Then as you exhale through the right nose send the energy to the spleen center and then you will see how the spleen center is glowing. Hold it there for six seconds then exhale. Repeat this process ten times. This exercise will help in energizing the Spleen *chakra*. Since spleen center is situated on the digestive system it will increase the vitality of our digestive system.

The next step is to raise the breath to the solar plex center. Imagine again that the white sunlight is entering slowly with your breath through the right nose with left nose closed, and hold the breath at the base center for ten seconds then as you exhale it raises the energy level to one count to spleen center. Hold it there for ten seconds then raise this energy one count to the solar plex center. Hold it there for ten seconds and then exhale the rest energy. Repeat this process ten times so that the solar plex is energized. When the solar plex is energized we will feel lightness and our body cells will start replicating with full vigour. We can repeat the same process with the heart center.

Imagine that we draw white light energy through our right nose with the left nose closed. Imagine that white light is at the base center and hold the breath for ten seconds then exhale it and raise the energy to one count to spleen center. Keep the energy there for ten seconds, then raise it to solar plex center by count of one and hold the energy there for ten seconds. Now raise the energy to heart center with count of one and hold the breath at heart center for ten seconds. At this time we will experience a flow of love at the heart and we see our heart will glow like a light. Then exhale the remaining breath. Repeat this process again ten times.

Throat Chakra

We can repeat the same process with throat *chakra*.

Imagine that we draw white light energy through our right nose with the left nose closed. Imagine that white light is at the base center. Hold the breath for ten seconds, then exhale it and raise the energy to one count to spleen center. Keep the energy there for ten seconds then raise it to solar plex center by count of one and hold the energy there for ten seconds. Now raise the energy to heart center with count of one and hold the breath at heart center for ten seconds. Now, raise the energy level to throat *chakra* by count of one and hold the breath at throat *chakra* for ten seconds and experience a glow at this center. The glow of the throat *chakra* gives energy to the vocal chords and this will help us in communicating with powerful force. Repeat this process again for ten times.

process again for ten times.

Brow Chakra

We can repeat the same process with Brow *chakra.*

Imagine that we draw white light energy through our right nose with left nose closed and imagine that white light is at the base center and hold the breath for 10 seconds, then exhale it and raise the energy to 1 count to spleen center. Keep the energy there for 10 seconds, then raise it to solar plex center by count of one and hold the energy there for 10 seconds. Then raise the energy to heart center with count of 1 and hold the breath at heart center for 10 seconds. Now, raise the energy level to throat *chakra* by count of 1 and hold the breath at throat *chakra* for 10 seconds. Then raise the energy to the brow *chakra* and hold the energy for more than 10 seconds and experience a glow at this center. When fully developed brow *chakra* enables to see various sorts of waking visions of people and places. People who are clairvoyant have powerful brow *chakra.* Repeat this process again ten times.

Crown *Chakra*

We can repeat the same process with crown *chakra.*

Imagine that we draw white light energy through our right nose with the left nose closed and imagine that white light is at the base center and hold the breath for 10 seconds, then exhale it and raise the energy to 1 count to spleen center. Keep the energy there for 10 seconds, then raise it tc solar plex center by count of one and hold the energy there for 10 seconds. Then raise the energy to heart center with count of 1 and hold the breath at heart center for 10 seconds.

Now, raise the energy level to throat *chakra* by count of 1 and hold the breath at throat *chakra* for 10 seconds. Then raise the energy to the brow *chakra* and hold the energy for more than 10 seconds and experience a glow at this center. Now, raise the energy to crown *chakra* by count of 1 and hold the energy there for 15 seconds. When fully developed crown *chakra* helps us to achieve an out of body experience. We will see unity of all lives.

Repeat this exercise 3 times and experience how you feel.

Meditation of Colours for Reviving *Chakras*

Sit cross-legged on a hard cushion carpet with your back and neck straight. It is essential to have the back and neck straight, as this will give us good concentration, as the spine is free and the body balanced on the two pelvic bones. Visualize that red light is radiating from base center. After 30 seconds imagine that red light is travelling upwards and starts radiating from backside, front side, right and left sides. Visualize further that red light is going upwards and downwards. After 30 seconds of visualization imagine that red light now becomes white and hold this image for 30 seconds.

Sitting in the above posture visualize that violet light is radiating from spine center. After 30 seconds imagine that violet light is travelling upwards and starts radiating from the backside, front side, right and left sides. Visualize further that violet light is going upwards and downwards. After 30 seconds of visualization imagine that violet light now becomes white and hold this image for 30 seconds.

Repeat this sequence in each of other centers.

Navel Center or Solar plexus	Green Color
Heart Center	Yellow-gold
Throat *Chakra*	Blue
Brow *Chakra*	Indigo
Crown *Chakra*	Purple

Each time, after radiating the particular colour in all directions let that colour become white light. All these postures of colours cause the *pranic* current to circulate vigorously. With practice of meditation beside powerful *chakras* we will gain devotion, cheerfulness, steadiness, patience, perseverance, courage, unselfishness, compassion and generosity. With the increasing purity, steadiness and one-pointedness of the heart and mind we become attuned to something of that supreme beauty which shines all over the world.

Summary of *Chakras* Power

Root *Chakra*

Location Base of Spine. Red Orange colour, powerful

creative energy, latent and potent serpent power, ready to shoot off.

Spleen Center. It has pink colour. It protects us from anxiety, toxicity and infection.

It is located halfway between pubis and navel.

Navel or Solar Plexus. Location just above the novel.

It is fire center for emotions, its colour is green and it is source of ambition.

Heart Chakra. Location just on the center of the heart.

Its colour is yellow. It is a source of compassion, the snake serpent fire transforms emotions into golden sun of love.

Throat Chakra. Location middle of the throat.

It has a blue colour like the sky. It is center of self expression and it also produces elation and source of divine communication.

Brow Chakras. Location middle of the forehead.

Its colour is indigo. It is center of extrasensory perception and intuition. It opens the third eye, then we have power of ecstatic vision and soul realization.

Crown Chakra. Location top of the head.

Its colour is purple.

It is source of absolute unity, silence, bliss, and opens the reality beyond duality, space and external. It empowers us with knowledge.

8

Obstruction to Concentration

Mind is hard to curb. It jumps like a monkey. Lord Krishna said in Gita "Mind is difficult to control". It is like a powerful wind which blows so fast that it drives away any object. Since mind is difficult to control it can be slowed down by constant practice of Yoga. Mind is like a magnet, attracting and repelling, and by the nature of its attraction we can determine repulsions. If we watch the thoughts, which come into our minds, we shall find that they are of the same kinds which we habitually encourage. The mind attracts the thoughts which are congruous with its normal activities.

If we, then, for a time, deliberately practise selection, the mind will soon do this selection for itself on the lines laid down for it, so that evil thoughts will not penetrate into the mind, while the good will ever find an open door.

The habit of concentration will strengthen the mind. Thoughts which are coming from outside should be diverted to good thinking. Bad thoughts, which have entered the mind, should be replaced with good thoughts: Never try to resist with the bad thoughts, simply replace the bad thoughts with good thoughts, the bad thoughts will simply drop away.

The mind behaves in rules of receptivity; the mind responds to its constitution; its answer to all.

At the initial stage the mind is positive towards evil and negative towards good, but by constant practice of good thinking we can make it positive towards good and negative towards bad or evil. We must think of that which we desire to receive, and refuse to think of that which we desire not to receive. Such a mind, in the Thought Ocean, which surrounds it, draws to itself the good thoughts, repels the evil, and thus ever grows purer and stronger amid the very thought conditions, which render another fuller and weaker.

The method of replacing one thought by another is one that may utilize to great advantage in many ways. If an unkind thought about another person enters the mind, it should at once be replaced by some virtuous thought, or some good action thought.

If the mind is harassed by anxiety, turn it towards peaceful thoughts that run through the life, the good law that will cover all things. This way anxiety will turn into subtle energy of peace.

It is a good plan constantly to furnish the mind with some high thoughts, some words of cheer, and some inspiration to noble thinking. Some words like in the Gayatri Mantra should be chanted in the morning. This will help to engage the mind again and again, during the day, and will be found repeating itself in the mind, whenever the mind is disengaged,

Meditation cannot be effectively performed until concentrations, at least partially, are mastered. It is difficult for a person to do meditation if his mind jumps like a monkey. First of all one should use the technique of concentration to arrest the jumping mind. For concentration is not an end, but means to an end.

It fashions the mind into an instrument which can be used at the will of the owner. When the concentration is directed to any object, with a view of piercing the veil, and reaching the life, and drawing that life into union with the life to which the mind belongs—then meditation is performed.

Concentration might be regarded as the shaping of the organ, meditation as its exercise.

The mind has been made one-pointed; it is then directed to and dwells steadily on any object of which knowledge is desired. By constant practice one can pierce the veil of ignorance on any object. Any one who desires to lead a spiritual and powerful life must devote some time to meditation. As soon the physical body can be sustained without food it becomes weak and careless, similarly spiritual body without meditation becomes weak and useless.

Only if the mind concentrates steady, and shuts out from the world, will the divine revel in it. God shows himself in his universe in endless forms, but within the human heart all the forms are dissolved and one will find steady peace inside the heart which is a fragment of peace like a God. In that silence, peace, strength and force flow into the soul, and the man of meditation is ever the most efficient man of the world.

The concentrated intelligence, the power of withdrawing outside the turmoil, means immensely increased energy at work, and denotes steadiness, self control and serenity.

The man of meditation is the man who wastes no time, scatters no energy, and misses no opportunity.

Such a man governs events. Because within him is the power whereof events are only the outer expression. He shares the divine life, and therefore divine power.

Everything is energy. Everything vibrates at its own level of reality, and while form appears to be solid, a simple examination under a microscope reveals that a solid object is actually alive with dancing molecules, vibrating with high speed, but appearing to us to be solid. Energy is a part of the stuff. So is the thought the part of energy. If that thought from energy is directed towards peaceful channel then every atom of our body will emit energy.

Physicists have proved that thought is a form of energy. Previously energy comprised of gravitation, electrical energy, weak and high electrical energy, and now thought has been included as a form of energy. So when you are having a thought about something that you would like to see happen for yourself, remember it is nothing more than connecting the two frequencies together to make the reality happen to you.

Keep in mind that if you are capable of conceiving the idea in your head as an image of something that you would like, then it is already there. Albert Einstein says, "Great spirits have always encountered violent opposition from mediocre minds. The other poster is made up solely of words. I am grateful to all those people who said no. It is because of them I find myself in Great thoughts."

Inherent within this third principle of visualization is the notion of openness. When you are willing to do whatever is necessary to formalize your images your thoughts will be open for all possibilities available to us.

Robert Fritz said :

"The way you activate the seeds of your creation is by making choices about the results you want to create. When you make a choice, you mobilize vast human energies and resources which otherwise go untapped." "All too often people fail to focus their choices upon results and, therefore, their choices are ineffective. If you limit your choices only to what seems possible or reasonable, you disconnect yourself from what you truly want and all that is left is a compromise."

Emerson said :

"The ancestor of every action is a thought. When we project our dreams into positive future, we see that we can have what we want. A positive image of the future not only shows us how to get there; it draws us to it, attracting us towards our dreams like a magnet."

The Sanctuary

Sanctuary is a place of retreat you build in your mind. Many people build sanctuary homes for retreating during summer times. Similarly, sanctuary build up in mind is the resting place of mind.

There are absolutely no limits to our sanctuary, although it is a good idea to put some limits on it. In this way, the sanctuary is a transitional point between the limitations of our physical existence and is unlimited. Mind is a great place of turmoil. Any outside disturbance can cause disturbance in mind. It is essential to calm our mind. Our mind can only be peaceful if we are unattached with the result of our actions. Attachment in the work will generate anger if we fail in our action. So the foremost condition to have a sanctuary of mind is to do work without attachment of result.

The White Light

Each time we enter our sanctuary, i.e., when our mind is peaceful then think that a pure white light cascades over us, which will be protecting and healing us. It surrounded us from all sides, and it is good for all concerned.

By practice of meditation this light can cascade into health center *chakras* and we can focus tremendous energy into them, and get lot of energy out of them.

The *chakras* are staffed with most competent health practitioners meditation can buy. These are most healing powers where anyone can buy.

Henry Ford said :

"I am looking for a lot of men who have an infinite capacity to not know what can't be done."

9

Benefits of Developing Your *Chakras*

Stress and Fertility Problems

People who are sick and have problems with their physical body can be greatly benefited by meditation and developing an inner peace.

Doctors did research that infertility can be cured to some extent by meditation and developing inner power. Infertility has affected some 10 million American couples. These couples have lost the ability to conceive due to some factor which is beyond their control.

Scientists have only recently pieced together the links between stress and fertility problems.

People who are stressed can disrupt the sequence of events, and block the flow of hormones, which are released by the brain and pituitary glands. Nerve fibres travelling in our body through the spinal cord also link the brain directly to the ovaries, uterus, and fallopian tubes. These connections are easy target of stress to enter and disrupt and interfere with conception—for example, by disrupting ovulation or having an adverse effect on pregnancy. Because of this similar links have been found between the brain and reproductive organs. In some men stress can reduce the sex drive and cause impotence.

Because infertility itself often causes enormous stress, a vicious cycle can easily occur. Infertile couples are deprived of having a child. This type of stress of dealing with infertility may worsen the physiological problem. Under the stress of infertility, a relationship can crumble.

The couple may no longer have much affection within their relationship. Their sexual life and family life may crumble. It is essential that infertile couples should be relieved of such turmoil. The question relevant is: will stress reduction help them to conceive?

In one study, doctors enrolled 54 women in a behavioural treatment programme. In ten weekly meetings, they were taught to do the meditation and relaxation. The response in the meeting as well as to practice at home meditation way for 20 minutes twice a day. By the end of the programme it was surprising to find they were significantly less anxious, depressed, and fatigued than before.

In addition, 34 per cent of these women became pregnant within six months of completing the programme. Women who had been infertile for a relatively short time had a significantly higher rate of conception than those who were infertile for longer period. This clearly proved that meditation, which reduces stress, could cure to some extent there infertility.

What can we say from this? The conception rate of 34 per cent within the group in six months was higher than is typical among other women who are not under treatment for infertility using meditation and stress reduction techniques. This clearly proves that stress reduction techniques may have been partially responsible of increasing fertility. In any case, relaxation or meditation training clearly contributed to peace of mind something beside their fertility, which is quite valuable in its own place in life. It leads to a significant improvement in emotional well-being and thus in the quality of life.

Yoga, or the meditation programme helped couples to conceive. It may have been by eliminating the vicious circle of stress and infertility, each intensifying and destroying the health of a person. Yoga could have helped in calming down the mind, which, in turn, had a great impact on the health of a person. The stress control by Yoga seems to have helped in gaining the lost control of their brain and mind.

Stress Control and Diabetese

Diabetese means excessive sweet urine. The sweetness comes from glucose, a sugar that is a major source of energy for the body's cells. When glucose cannot enter in the cell then that glucose enters in the urine and it flows with urine and it is one of the signs of diabetes. Normally, glucose enters the cells from the bloodstream with the help of hormone insulin, secreted by the pancreas. In the case of diabetes, glucose cannot readily enter in the cells. When glucose is unable to enter in the cells then cells are deprived of the energy that is created by glucose. This later harms eye cells and a person becomes blind.

Whereas the glucose accumulates in the bloodstream, and when it exceeds a certain level it spills over to the urine. People who are diabetic their blood sugar is high. This sometimes causes kidney failure if the disease is not treated in time.

There are two major types of diabetes, Type I, or insulin-dependent: this type of diabetes affects one million Americans apart from being present in people all over the world. It generally develops at childhood and it is hereditary.

In Type II diabetes, insulin is produced, but defects in a body cells make them resistant to the insulin and they do not allow the insulin to enter inside. Even when they are exposed to the hormones, they cannot make insulin normally. Those with Type II diabetes are rapidly having an increase in this country. More than eight million Americans now have diabetes, four million of whom are undiagnosed.

It is possible to medicinally treat diabetics. Type I diabetes can be cured by the injection of insulin, whereas type II diabetes can be cured by exercise, dieting, and some minor medicines. For both types of diabetics, however, stress control through meditation may also play a key role in keeping sugar levels in check. Evidence of a biochemical link between diabetes and high stress levels was found at Harvard Medical School in 1970. At extreme stress conditions, stress hormones called adrenaline and cortisol, are produced by the adrenal gland. Doctors noted cats that had been frightened by the presence of a dog passed sugar in their urine which is a symptom of diabetes.

Why did stress produce this reaction? Doctors found that at times of heightened anxiety, large quantities of stress hormones are released into the blood by the adrenal glands. This causes an increase in the blood sugar.

Duke University experimented with 12 patients with high Type II diabetes and high levels of stress. For nine days, the patients remained at Duke University hospital. Half of them received progressive meditation training and EMG (electromyographic) biofeedback along with an exercise regimen whereas the other half received only diet and exercise.

At the end of the experiment, the patients who were taught meditation showed better metabolic control than the others did. Their blood sugar was low compared to the other group.

We should learn more about how stress affects diabetes control and how techniques to control stress can be useful in reducing the effects of the disease. One useful new advance for diabetics is the development of techniques to learn to recognize when blood sugar is high or low.

Psychologist Daniel Cox and his colleagues at the University of Virginia have designed a method that allows us to relate our feelings, stress, and sensations to blood sugar levels.

High blood sugar has a correlation with high stress and emotions. High levels of stress have physiological effects that influence glucose metabolism and can increase our blood sugar level, making diabetes more difficult to control. Whereas, by meditation when stress is reduced, they found that blood sugar level is lowered.

Arthritis can be Cured by Meditation

Psycho-analyst Franz Alexander and his colleagues theorized that individuals who repress anger and are unable to express emotions were particularly likely to develop ailments like arthritis. People with rheumatoid arthritis have been identified as having emotional problems on the screen. While these notions about the psychological roots of arthritis have provided only limited advances, other approaches may provide important insights into the link between psychological states and the severity of arthritis. Many doctors at the Duke University did apply the group of arthritis patients to meditation techniques and found those patients arthritis pain reduced.

Sense of Coherence

A person's attitude toward life, too, may have a significant impact on his/her ability to deal with arthritis. People who score high on sense of coherence tests feel that their circumstances make sense and what is more, that life makes sense. You can develop a sense of coherence by doing meditation and Yoga. We can also develop coherence by positive thinking.

Healing through Imagery

A wide range of conditions including chronic pain, allergies, high blood pressure, irregular heartbeats, cold and flu symptoms, stress-related gastrointestinal and urinary complaints can be cured by concentration and imagery practice and transcendental meditation.

Many of these benefits stem directly from the relaxing effects of imagery and meditation. In fact, the most common, most useful, and easiest application of imagery in health care is its use in relaxation and stress reduction. Imagery is a simple exercise :

Keep your eyes closed while you take a few deep, easy breaths, focus your mind on some beautiful scenic place like a mountain with green trees and flowing streams of water falling. Concentrate on this scenery for a few minutes and imagine you are walking across that mountain and concentrate on beautiful flower tree, which you come across. Focus intently on the sights, smells, and physical sensations associated with that event. You will feel relaxed, your mind flow will slow down, you will feel calmer and more alert, refreshed as well as have a new-found sense of energy.

In many cases, imagery may have beneficial effects on patients even though its effects on their particular diseases cannot be determined. Another role imagery has in medical care is to put one in touch with their feelings about their illness. Imagery can be helpful in almost any medical situation that requires problem solving and decision making. Receptive imagery treatment may involve a dialogue with images representing symptoms or the illness. In most experiences, this two-way use of imagery to spur communication between mind and body yields the most profound healing responses.

What does it Cost?

Mind/body approaches are generally inexpensive. It costs

next to nothing. Furthermore, to learn the meditation and relaxation response costs nothing. You cannot get good returns only by simply using your time wisely.

Anyone thinking of trying a fee-based approach will naturally want to know how much of the cost is covered by medical insurance. You can pay thousands of dollars on these treatments and still not get 100 per cent satisfaction. With the mind/body approach you can relax and reduce the impact of those diseases to a minimum. If the mind/body treatment is used all over the country it can greatly reduce medical costs and help in reducing the huge federal deficit.

The government, instead of opening thousands of hospitals and medical schools, can push these meditative techniques and gain in controlling huge medical investments in the future.

United States is investing about 12 per cent of its GNP in medical treatment. Its investment in medical science is the highest in the world. In spite of such a huge investment, there are about 40 million Americans who do not have any medical insurance. Among so many others, Medicare and insurance rates are rising and benefits are declining.

In these critical situations, it is best to use mind/body techniques, which are less costly and can be used without opening hospitals.

In general mind/body meditation approaches have shown great potential for improving the quality of life and reducing the pain and difficulty of symptoms for people with various chronic diseases. They may help control or reverse certain underlying disease processes. By reducing the effects of stress, they may help to prevent diseases from developing. The physical and emotional risk of using these techniques is minimal, while their potential benefit is high. The economic cost of mind/body approaches is low. These techniques can easily be applied in the context of conventional medicine, instead of being seen as anti-thetical to it.

Informed consumers who want to try a meditation approach often want answers to a number of questions that their doctors may not able to help them with.

It is now an indisputable fact, however, that the mind can influence the body and that there is a precise nature of a linkage between the mind and body. There is a more real debate over whether and how the mind/body connection can be harnessed to help people stay well or recover from illness.

Apart from being widely recognised all over the world effective and responsible mind/body approaches are beginning to be used widely in university and private clinics, in hospitals, and by corporations in U.S.A. (i.e., AT & T, Johnson & Johnson, IBM, and General Motors.)

Chronic Pain : A New Way to Control it with Meditation

Some 10 to 30 per cent of Americans suffer from some degree of pain in their daily life. In some cases, the pain is so acute that it becomes an unbearable burden. Such chronic pain can last for months or even for years at a time thus having a tremendously damaging effect on the quality of life. Its damaging effects on the immune system can easily see pain's direct affect on one's physical life.

Society pays a high cost for chronic pain, as more than 11.7 million Americans are in its grip. About 550 million workdays are lost in this country due to chronic pain. According to recent estimates, the costs in disability compensation and loss productivity may be as high as $100 billion annually.

When pain cannot be rectified people often feel abandoned by the medical community as well as angered by the bills for treatments that were not effective. In such situations, much frustration can be caused.

The Gate Control Theory: Currently, many researchers subscribe to the gate control theory. Psychologist Ronald Melzack developed this theory in 1965. Melzack suggested that there is a gating system in the central nervous system that opens and closes to let in or block pain messages through the brain. A person's emotional state and the way he/she interprets a situation can both open and close gates.

The Path to Pain: According to the gate theory of pain, your thoughts, beliefs and emotions may affect how much pain you feel from a given physical sensation.

First, sensory messages travel from stimulated nerves to the spinal cord—the body's pain highway. There, they are reprocessed and sent through open gates to the thalamus; the brain's depot for tactile information. Once the nerve signals reach the brain, the sensory information is processed in the context of the individual's current mood, state of attention, and their prior experience. If the brain sends a message back down to close the gate, the pain signals to the brain are blocked. If the brain orders the pain gates to open wider, the pain signals intensify.

How does this happen? For one thing, thoughts and emotions can directly influence responses, including muscle tension, blood flow, and the level of brain chemicals—all of which play important roles in the production of pain. Psychological factors can indirectly influence pain by the way you cope with it. Anticipating pain before it strikes, for example, can worsen the situation.

Perhaps the most common and useful techniques for controlling pain are muscle relaxation. It decreases muscle spasms, reduces and controls muscle tension, and helps control other physiological mechanisms involved in nervous system arousal and pain production. In the relaxation method, meditation and the use of imagery are used to eliminate the pain.

A recent review of several studies conducted by Ohio State University found that relaxation training alone, on average, produced a 45 per cent improvement for those with tension headaches, and 30 per cent improvement of migraine headaches.

Stress Control and Heart Attack

The coronary arteries—so named because they encircle the heart like a crown—supply heart muscles with the blood they need to function over time. Cholesterol and other substances can accumulate to form a plaque, a deposit in the wall of the artery. If a blood clot then blocks that passageway, it can choke off the blood supply to the heart muscle and cause a heart attack. It is found that people having high stress as a result of hostility increase their blood pressure due to the increase in adrenaline and cortisol hormones.

These hormones raised in blood pressure, make the blood clot more rapidly and accelerate the growth of atherosclerotic plaques-deposits in blood within the blood vessels that clog the coronary arteries.

The fact that hostile people have higher than normal increases in blood pressure and stress hormones when they are annoyed or angry shows that they have a low threshold for triggering the sympathetic nervous system.

In addition, hostile people are slower than others to activate the parasympathetic nervous system—the part that can protect the body from the onslaught of stress hormones. A high level of blood cholesterol is a major indicator of a heart attack.

Meditation can help in reducing a heart attack. Your stress is caused by fear generated in the mind. That fear might be any thing : it might be loosing a job, getting a divorce, being killed in a plane crash (death is, incidentally, the most widespread fear), loosing money in business or any myriad of other possibilities. All these fears are generated in the mind.

Thoughts that are roaming in the mind are a creator of all our fears—thoughts from the past, present, and future. So the way to eliminate fear and reduce stress is to get rid of thoughts. If the flow of thoughts is trickled down to a minimum then fear will be gone which will then result in reducing the stress.

Meditation or the chanting of *mantras* can only eliminate thoughts. It has been found that meditation will slow down the thoughts and lower blood pressure. Research done by Harvard Medical School shows that high blood pressure and stress hormones can be reduced by doing relaxation's and transcendental meditation.

Fortunately, there are ways to diminish the negative health effects of stress which can be countered with a commitment to change, to learn to control your stress by meditation. Meditation can improve the prognosis for heart patients, and help healthy people prevent heart disease as well.

Cancer Control through Meditation

When people ponder whether psychological factors can lead

to tumors. Stress, beliefs, and emotions can affect lifestyle choices and health related behaviour.

According to widely accepted theory of cancer the immune surveillance hypothesis, the immune system plays a constant, ongoing role in preventing cancer from developing. This theory holds that cancer cells are always developing spontaneously in the body, but the immune system's ability to recognize them as abnormal and destroy them generally prevents them from developing into tumors. Natural killer cells are thought to play a key role in attacking cancer. It is only when the number of cancer cells become too great to be destroyed or when the natural killer cells are suppressed or inactive that cancer develops.

If this theory is true, and if emotional stress can weaken the immune system considerably, then link between the mind and cancer causation would be theoretically plausible.

One interesting set of experiments, done by psychologist Martin Seligman and his colleagues at the university of Pennsylvania subject to two groups of mice.

One group of mice was subjected to stress by giving them electric shocks, whereas another group was not subjected to stress. Now, they injected tumor injection to both groups of mice, mice which were subjected to stress shocks tumors develop much faster whereas group which were not subjected to stress shocks cancer spread at much slower speed. This experiment showed that mice stressed in different ways had higher levels of the stress hormone cortisol and experienced immune suppression.

Despite a lack of scientific evidence for its physical benefits, active or guided meditation has become a popular way to put the mind to work to battle cancer. It clearly helps some patients psychologically to gain a sense of control and doing something.

Although such meditation may reduce the patient's sense of helplessness a benefit that in it can enhance health.

The problem with these treatments comes when patients whose health does not improve believe they failed and become depressed because they feel they are not strong enough mentally to cure or control their cancer.

For many people, spiritual, philosophical, or religious beliefs are central to coping with cancer and help them find meaning in having the disease. Usually, these beliefs include the existence of a higher power of conviction that life has order and meaning beyond our rational everyday perceptions. Calling on a higher power for help can bring great solace during illness, but no one yet knows whether spiritual beliefs have an impact on survival.

Relaxation, guided imagery, hypnosis, biofeedback, meditation, distraction and other behavioural techniques can help people cope with the side effects of treatment for cancer.

AIDS Control through Meditation

Our aim is to help these men face one of the most disturbing diagnoses in medicine—being HIV positive. The stress management programme that is offered to these types of people is physical relaxation and exercise to help calm both bodies and mind.

Doctors use this psychological support system to achieve physiological benefits, specifically by bolstering the immune system. If a stress management programme could offer medical improvement to people facing illness as dire as AIDS, it might be promising for patients struggling with countless other difficulties as well.

In general, HIV infection damages the body by attacking components of the immune system, most notably helper T cells, that identify and attack viruses.

Eventually, as these and other cells become ravaged, the immune system becomes so compromised that the body is left vulnerable to a host of life threatening infections and rapidly progressing cancers at which point the patient is considered to have AIDS.

Research has shown sense of lack of control over life, social isolation, and depression caused decline in immune system cells, including helper T cells. It has been found that improving the psychological health of patients with HIV infection would help their physical health by strengthening the immune system. It was observed that in early stages of infection stress management programmes helped.

Stress management programmes was tested for HIV infected patients. It was found that benefit for stress management programme still holds good. It appears that stress management affects the immune system for the better—both during an acute stress attack on learning of the deadly infection and the early adjustment period afterwards.

Other researchers are now finding that depression is linked to the progression of HIV infection. The University of California, San Francisco, followed 330 HIV-positive men for over six years. It was reported that the AIDS men, who fall in grip of stress destroy their T cells fast, and develop Aíds sooner, and had twice the mortality rate of non-depressed two groups.

Study has shown the possibility that treating depression could slow down the decline of the immune system in HIV-positive people.

Group stress management programme for people with chronic illnesses are becoming a common mind/body treatment. Research has long shown that such groups are extremely effective way of teaching people more successful ways to shoulder the psychological burden their illness causes. And recent research on gay men infected with AIDS virus adds evidence that these groups can offer physiological benefits as well.

Healing of the Weak by the Strong through a Trained Healer

It has been proved that man having a vigorous health and spiritual advancement is throwing off vital energy, which may be absorbed by others. In this way the receiver of the energy can get strengthened, and some minor illnesses can be cured.

As we have discussed before *Prana* is the source of energy. If that energy is directed towards a patient who is sick and who is depleted of strength, it can benefit the patient and he can recover from the illness.

The healing of the weak by the strong may thus be achieved, in certain cases, merely by physical proximity, which may be unconscious and automatic.

Much benefit may often be given merely by pouring into the patient's system with vitalizing energy; merely increase the circulation of *Prana* in some other body that will cure some minor illness. Headaches are usually caused by congestion, either of blood or the vital fluid, sometimes called magnetism. A strong current of energy directed to the patient will wash away the congested matter and headache will disappear.

Healing can be improved considerably if the healer has knowledge of Anatomy and Physiology; in that case he can make a mental image of a diseased organ, and image it as it is good health. The strong thought can change the defective cells into healthy cells.

Healthy and methodical way of healing is as follows : The patient assumes a comfortable position either sitting or lying down, and is instructed to relax completely.

A healer then passes with his hands over the patient's body or over that portion of it which is affected by the disease. After each pass the healer must take care to throw off from himself the etheric matter he has withdrawn, otherwise some of them remain in own system and may harm him latter.

Usually, it is sufficient to jerk the hands sharply downwards and away from oneself, or the magnetism may be thrown into basin of water, the water will wash, the curse may be removed. The process may be assisted after this preliminary portion of the treatment is completed. The next stage is to pour into the patient one's own magnetic fluid and *prana*. This is done by making similar passes, though this time with strong effort of will to pour out one's own force into the patient. This is as before may be done by means of long sweeping passes over the whole body or some special area.

It should be noted that the healer should be in perfect health, because otherwise he is liable to pour into patient some of his own unhealthy magnetism.

It should be noted that in magnetic healing clothing is somewhat of a barrier, silk being in this respect worst. Patient should wear minimum resistance clothes.

Generally speaking, it may be said that anything, which promotes health also, reacts favourably on the higher vehicles. Unused muscles, for example, not only tend to deteriorate but produce a congestion of magnetism. This means a week place in the etheric double, through which unpleasant germs, such as those of infection, may enter.

Similarly, mental or astral ill health will almost surely, sooner or later, be reflected as physical disease.

So, a person should take extra precaution in healing processes.

Oxytocins and Endorphins: The Positive Forces of Love

Love is central to human existence. Without love human life will become dull and devastating. Now researchers are beginning to sort and find that mind and brain work together and produce a wild tender love force in our body. The force of love is called Oxytocin which is a binding force which binds mother and child together.

It fuels romantic love also. Oxytocin also acts like a neurotransmitter, or chemical messenger that can guide behaviour without which a cow cannot recognize her own calf. Oxytocin has a big impact on mothers; it induces openness and devotion for their child. As child sucks the mother's milk the level of oxytocin rises in mother's body. Mothers with higher levels of oxytocin are more sensitive to other people's feelings and better understanding of non-verbal communication.

This also proves that oxytocin bind to centers in the brain involved with emotion. Oxytocin also acts like a tranquilizer, lowering a new mother's blood pressure.

Love's other messengers in the brain are endorphins, or brain opiates, which body produces itself all the time. High level of brain opiates kills pain and induces a state of happiness and relaxation.

Inverse of love is hate or grief. In a state of pain and grief endorphin level is kicked out by the same brain cells.

Researchers have shown that passionate or platonic love affects the whole body, setting the heart pounding, making the stomach do flip flops, and igniting the fire in the body. It opens the most of the *chakras* mouths and set them to vibration. Researchers said these sensations are the work of a vagus nerve, which travels a zigzag path in a body, coordinating the activities of internal organs.

These vagus ferries signals between our innards and our brains conveying information upward about our internal state and sending orders down from brain to the heart, the stomach, the lungs and the sex organs.

These flow of forces also play a major part in sex reproduction and people who can utilize these forces can benefit much whereas people who misuse these forces loose their vitality and harm themselves.

If we channel the flow of river for irrigation it will enhance food production, whereas if it is used for dump dirts it will poison the whole water.

These forces which are travelling inside the body help slow the heart and keep the body calm and enough for the brain to pay attention to emotional signals from other people.

It is correct to say that the heart speaks the language of love. Where love is strengthened hope is restored.

The Importance of Knowing Yourself

Krishnamurti, a great philosopher, said you may have all the academic degrees in the world, but if you do not know yourself you are the most stupid person. To know oneself is the very purpose of all education. Without self-knowledge, merely to gather facts or take notes so that you can pass examination does no good. You may quote *Bible*, *Koran*, or *Gita*, but unless you know yourself you are like a parrot repeating words.

Whereas the moment you begin to know yourself, however little there sets in an extraordinary process of creativeness. It is discovery to suddenly see yourself as you actually are : greedy, quarrelsome, angry, envious, stupid. To see the fact without trying to alter it, just to see exactly what you are is an astonishing revelation. From there you can go deeper and deeper, infinitely, because there is no end to self-knowledge.

Through self-knowledge you begin to find out what is God, what is truth, what is that state which is timeless. Your teacher may pass on to you the knowledge which he received from his teacher, and you may do well in your examination; but, without knowing yourself all other knowledge has very little meaning.

That is why it is important for the educator to be educated in the true sense of the word, which means that he must know the workings of his own mind and heart, see himself exactly as he is in the mirror of relationship. Self-knowledge is the beginning of wisdom.

In self-knowledge is the whole universe, it embraces all the struggles of humanity.

Srimad Bhagavatam said that :

> One should be situated in the transcendental position, beyond the stages of material consciousness, and should be aloof from all other conceptions of life. Thus realizing freedom from false ego, one should see his own self just as he sees the sun in the sky.

When we say that give up our ego, this means that we give up our false ego, but real ego is always present. In the conditioned state, one accepts everything as an object of sense gratification, and in the liberated state one accepts everything for the sake of the true inner self.

10

Senses and the Healing of Emotions

Researchers are discovering the importance of senses in healing, emotions and well-being of man. Growing evidences have been gathered that people who ignored senses can fall prey to diseases in physical, and emotional levels. Beyond their capacity to heal and delight, the senses have also opened a window on the working of the human brain. The senses of hearing, sight, smell and touch give solid evidence how the brain works. As the brain has trillions of neurons each has hardwired connection, which makes it, one of the largest neutral circuits in the universe.

Previously, it was assumed that sense organs did most of the processing of information about the world, but now researchers have found that senses are just stations that transmit the signals, whereas all the signals are processed by brain.

Sight

Vision has offered scientists their most powerful insight on how the brain works. While we perceive a unified scene, the brain dissects the view into many parts, each of which triggers a different set of neurons, called visual map. One map responds to motion, another form responds to colour, third map responds to the form. There are five such maps in the visual system.

The brain also does much of the heavy lifting for colour vision, so much so that some people with brain damage see the world in shades of gray. Each person has a different palette. There are nine genes that control the colour. The permutations and combinations of these genes will encompass entire colour pattern of the world.

Hearing

Hearing is a gateway to language. In a normal child the ears tune themselves to human sounds soon after birth cementing the neural connections between language, emotions and intelligence. Hearing in the Veda is related with directions. Sound of each direction will tell the brain where to go. An inability to hear the sounds of human speech is called autism, which make children emotionally sick as they hear frightening voices.

Touch

The new view that a newly-born child who is given massage three times a day for 15 minutes will grow and gain more weight compared to babies who are put in a intensive care unit.

Being touched has a healing power. Massage, researchers have found, can ease the pain and boost the immune systems of AIDS patients.

A Swedish physiologist has found that gentle stroking can stimulate the body and release oxytocin, sometimes called the love hormone. There are deep connections between love and touching. Oxytocin also blunts pain and dampens the hormones released when a person is anxious or stressed.

Smell

According to Gary Beauchamp, Director of Philadelphia's Manual Chemical Senses Center, Odour a plays a very important role in human behaviour. Men can smell fire from far away and take precaution against it. Baby can smell its mother and stop crying. The sense of smell is the most celebrated capacity and very powerful to stir the memory. Hit a trip wire of smell and memories explode at once.

According to an article in the *News Week* Dr Herz, said that smells carry an emotional quality. An odour's first way station in the brain is the olfactory bulb which are, two blueberries-sized lumps of cortex from which neurons extend through the skull into a nose. Smell molecules, those waiting off a cinnamon bun, for example, bind to these olfactory neurons, which fire off their signals first to the olfactory bulb and then to the limbic system- the seat of sexual drive. Connections between the olfactory bulb and neocortex or thinking part of the brain are secondary roads compared to the high ways leading to emotional centers.

Previously, scientists thought all smells were made up of combinations of seven basic odours. Now, scientist have found 1,000 genes corresponding to about 1,000 types of olfactory neurons in the nose. Each of these neuronal types respond to one and only one type of odour molecule. Brain can recognize about 10,000 different odours. El and Buck have now discovered that the olfactory bulb contains a map similar to those the brain employs for vision and hearing. The *chakra* sitting in the nose can stimulate the hearing and fill the nose with more power.

Taste

Taste is also an important sense organ. People like different tastes of different foods. Some like hot food and some like sweet food. All tongues are not created equal. How intense the flavours seem is determined by our heredity.

According to scientists you might be a non-taster, average taster, or a super taster. They found that super tasters are tending to be thinner and have lower cholesterol, whereas non-tasters tend to prefer sweets and fatty foods and are heavy weight.

Sight

Human senses detect only a fraction of reality. The eye can see only certain wave-length whereas there are many minute wave lengths the eye cannot detect and can only be detected through telescope or microscope.

Many people have to wear glasses just to see the normal vision. Our nose can detect only fraction of smell whereas dogs can detect thousand times more than man can.

We cannot see during night whereas an owl can see in darkness. We have limited ability of hearing whereas many birds and insects can hear much more than human-beings. Human-beings can see, feel, taste, touch and smell not the world, the once their brains have concocted. People imagine that they are seeing what really there, but they are actually not. The eyes take in the light reflected by objects around us, but the brain only pays attention to part of the scene. We can see only things which we focus our attention on we can ignore the others.

Chakra can enhance the powers of senses wherein we can see even in darkness, and smell 10 to power of 23 different types of smell. Imagine we can control our weight by being super tasters, and hear the lightest noise simulated by music. So by developing these *chakras* we can become super human-beings.

Interactions of Bodies

Each of the bodies existing in nature grow by use. The physical body grows through the exercise of its various faculties. Its use or abuse action or neglect, will raise or lower the quality and responsiveness of the bodies.

The effect of certain emotions has an adverse impact on astral as well as mental bodies. Note particularly that, as stated, it is not the spiritual man himself who gets angry, or feels depressed, or is fearful. Man fails to control his astral body due to which he suffered uncontrolled reactions due to outer disturbances. A careful analysis of the conditions of our consciousness at such a time will often, probably invariably, reveal that there is an inner voice, the voice of the Self, which is trying to diffuse the crises and is desperately trying to control the body and to bring it back to a condition of balance.

In many ways the astral body is drawn upward or downward and its present degree of unfoldment in any person is the balance sheet of all his efforts of the past, for good or bad.

Fortunately, an effort expended in the subtler kinds of matter, associated with the highest emotions or thoughts, produces more effect than a similar effort exerted in substances of grosser kind, just as a given amount of energy used to walk through the air with feet upon the ground, would result in a greater distance being covered than by an equivalent amount expended in an attempt to walk on the ocean bed through the water.

Gradually, by many such activities, the Self and its bodies are going forward on the pathway of life, each improving as time rolls by.

Functions Performed by the *Chakras*

Now that the subject of man's subtler bodies has been introduced we can consider some important *chakras* which play a vital role in man's physical self and evolution of human consciousness. Each *chakra* performs a dual function within the body. It absorbs life and energy and also acts as a transformer by means of which the vital forces generated within a body are changed in intensity so that they can be expressed through a denser vehicle, in precisely the same manner as electrical energy can be transformed from electrical potential to another.

Through the *chakra* we can reproduce emotional creations of the astral body within the physical. The physical atom vibrates in a physical environment in certain frequency. The astral forces of the *chakra* will intensify the vibration of physical atom or it might reduce the vibration of the atom in the physical. This same fact applies to any of the higher bodies in its relationship to the vehicles of consciousness lower or denser than itself.

In addition to the food we eat, and water we drink, the physical body absorbs forces from the etheric atmosphere, which surround us. One of these forces comes from the earth and is called *Kundalini*; the other comes from the Sun. It is called *Prana* or vitality. Neither of these has yet been recognized by science, though the latter seems to be suspected by some scientists.

Kundalini is the lowest level of expression and it is the densest. It affects the physical construction of the dense body. It affects our physical body and gives energy and vitality. Those who dig the soil and do some gardening know the feeling of well-being such an intimate contact with the soil can bring. This *Kundalini* force is absorbed by a root *chakra*, which is situated near the lower end of the spine and opens out at the surface of the etheric body. After absorption and internal action, the *kundalini* rises up the spine and is distributed throughout the nervous of the body. It also acts upon the blood stream and sex organs.

At the same time, the spleen *chakra* also receives another set of force which is called *Prana*. These *Prana* and *Kundalini* spread and are redistributed along the path of the nervous system and play an important role in man's higher level of consciousness.

Prana comes to us directly from the Sun. It is the active power in producing all vital phenomena. It is called the "Vitality Globule".

You can notice these particles when facing away from the sun and looking into a blue sky. This vitality globule or *prana* is absorbed by the spleen center. In the spleen center it is broken down into seven different colours like a spectrum as follows:

The blue and violet colours from the spleen are sent to the throat *chakra*. Two other colours red and orange, go to the root center. Yellow goes to the heart center. The green colour goes to the Navel center.

The seventh, rose colour is distributed throughout the entire nervous system.

While *Kundalini* and *Prana* are necessary for the physical well-being and vital activities of the dense physical body, it could not function without the forces, which come into it through the *chakras* from the Astral and Mental bodies. When these forces are withdrawn the physical body is robbed of their supporting influence and dies.

It is in the higher Mental and Spiritual worlds that man's greatest progress will be made as his evolution proceeds and, therefore, these two centers will assume a widening significance as time passes. There will come a time when the *Kundalini* will unfold its higher potencies and passing up the spine, it will stimulate all the centers into increased activity and continue on to produce far-reaching effects in the Brow and Crown *chakras*, endowing the man in his physical consciousness with the power to express spiritual manifestations far beyond anything hitherto accomplished.

The Physical and Spiritual Self

The *chakras* exist in each of the bodies, the centers, being coincidental, with the outermost parts stretching further because of the larger size of the subtler bodies. They perform similar functions though modified by the nature of the vehicle itself. However, each one is a transformer of force, the contiguous surfaces acting by induction to effect the transformation, exactly as the coils of an electrical transformer induce a current over a space without actual contact. Thus, in the physical world man's vehicles of consciousness are, as it were, welded into one and, though modified and limited by the transition. In the physical body man can express the whole range of consciousness that his several vehicles of consciousness cover.

The physical body appears to be same for ordinary man. Our senses tell us that it remains the same from day to day, but what the senses tell us is not true. The body does not remain the same day by day. It changes each day and in seven years entire cells of the body change. All the cells are made up of millions of cells, which are specialized in various functions. These cells grow, multiply and die.

Far from being a stable entity, the body is changing from moment to moment, cells are being born, others in equal numbers are dying and being eliminated from the system through the pores of the skin and the breath as it is exhaled from the lungs. The body which we had seven years ago undergoes a total change.

Our body is changing itself while we retain our identity unchanged from birth until death.

Not only does the spiritual man maintain his identity amid perpetual change, but he is the presiding genius which issues order to all its senses and provides them with food without which it can not survive. Huxley likened the body to a fountain, which maintains a continuity of outline, yet its parts do not remain the same for even a few seconds.

Another way in which we can survey this subject is to examine the essential nature of these things—the one material, the other spiritual. While cells of a body absorb oxygen, build protoplasm from food and help other cells to build the wonderful body. On the other hand, a spiritual self helps man to gain experience, develop wisdom from knowledge, make beneficial mental adaptations to changes in environment. The spiritual man also develops social and religious institutions by means of which he may meet with others in mental and religious harmony.

The ideas which have been presented here are, drawn from theosophical sources, regarding man and his bodies. They are claimed by some to be known as facts by direct observation. We can compare human expressions of love and hate, of bravery and fear, of inspiration and depression, that all the genius which is gradually conquering the universe itself, which has developed step by step in achievement over billions of years, arose without any kind of guidance whatsoever, by an infinitude of repetitions of purest chance, out of twenty simple chemical elements from which the very people who take such an incredible attitude have never succeeded in releasing anything more than energy of one kind to or another.

Our feelings, our thoughts, our imaginations, our desires, the physical body itself, will try to establish their identity with the reality within. When the outer voices are stilled and the search is carried deeply within, in silence and sincerity, the self can be found.

The Aura

"Aura" is a Latin word meaning "gently moving air", a breath of air, fragrance, "light" and glow light. The aura is an energy field, which surrounds the body and permeates it, like a kind of halo. It consists of the seven auras which belong to man's seven subtle energy bodies. Generally, a distinction is made between:

1. The spiritual aura which has a diameter of 15 to 18 feet.
2. The mental aura, which usually has a diameter of up to eight feet.
3. The etheric aura, which radiates from the physical body to a length of about eight inches.

Since the auras overlap, it is not possible to determine them individually. What clairvoyants usually see, however, is the etheric aura. This is perceived as being a kind of translucent field consisting of different colours and patterns. The aura can change in colour, size, structure and intensity according to the mental and emotional state of the person involved. Strongly felt emotions and physical and mental illness will be reflected by the appearance of aura.

In an analysis made by the British Colour Council, the aura was determined as possessing over 4,700 individually registered shades. Not only human beings but also plants, animals and stones have auras.

The fact that these fields of energy do not exist solely in the imagination of few people has been proved scientifically by Kirlian photography, a special method which makes the aura visible. This Kirlian photography is his so-called Energy Emission Analysis.

The strong auras are responsible for transferring the energy from one level of body to another. Since the auras interact among themselves, the higher spiritual energy entering from the crown *chakra* interacted with the mental aura and from it descended to etheric aura which transfer the energy to the physical body. When physical body receives such a tremendous energy that it energizes all the cells and that energy travels from head to leg. This energy acts like a Gamma ray and has the power of healing of our physical illness.

Science and Energy Fields

Researchers working in the areas of Biology and Physics have presented data that appears to substantiate the active existence of a biological energy field within living organisms. During 1940 Dr Harold and S. Burr of Yale University advanced their Electrodynamic Theory of Life. They used sensitive voltmeters and measured voltage gradients between different areas of human body. When the instruments are sensitive enough, the field can be detected even without skin contact. Burr and his co-workers found a characteristic field, what they termed "L" or life field, in every kind of living form they examined. In addition to this, they found that the L field was constant in its rhythmic pattern even after the molecules of an organism had been completely replaced by other molecules.

Increased DC electromagnetic flow was associated with feelings of well-being.

The body was seen to have a number of sub-fields of energy that interact with each other. Burr stated repeatedly that these were true energy fields. These fields were seen to be intimately connected to the organization of life.

The use of subtle consciousness in a "passive-volitional" mental framework was effective in altering various energy fields in the body. In this regard they said that to increase warmth in specific areas of the body by thought and imagery is a form of the thermal energy in the system. To change EEG patterns is to influence the electromagnetic field of the brain.

These fields can be understood in standard magnetic terms and quantitatively measured. A similar phenomenon is seen in acupuncture, used in the East for long time. The acupuncture theory identifies the Ki force of acupuncture with other energies.

Almost every human culture has made a similar energy and labelled this force or energy. Hebrews called it Ruach. The Congolese Elima. The American Indian called it Manitu and Sufi Baraka. The Burr work on L fields and the simpler biofeedback cases are empirical support for these organized fields and relationships in and around the body . Notice that Burr detected the field at some distance from the body.

The Bio-Gravitational Field

Research in the Soviet Union has also focused on this area. The general term used is bioplasm. Here it is noted that the spine appears to be the center of bioplasmic activity which is also called as "Prana".

This field is highly conducive and provides opportunities for the accumulation and transfer of energy within the organism as well as different organisms. Bioplasm is considered a fifth state of matter as explored and developed by rigorous technology.

This energy field has a dynamic behaviour that does not conform to our presently established laws of Biology and Physics. It is called bio-gravitational field. This bio-gravitational field is intimately connected with our emotional and cognitive life.

From certain data it can be inferred that bio-gravitational field arises in an organism as a consequence of changes in conformation of protein structures as a result of the transformations which occur with polypeptide molecules. This a body of plasma with its abundant ions, free electronics and free protons. This mechanism is operative since in each cell of our bodies, in any particular moment the protein molecules together with the layer of intercellular water adjacent to them are in coherent high frequency oscillatory states. In other words, the protein and water molecules in our bodies vibrate synchronously.

This bio-gravitational field of the organism as outlined above has certain properties in common with natural force. It has little power like gravitation. It can be detected and focused. It can be positive and negative and thus can cause attraction and repulsion. It can carry information. A field of such force can exist even without source.

Another scientist Dubrov has shown how these synchronous vibrations or levels lead to the increased generation of bio-gravitation of the bioplasmic field in the form of an "energy body". This energy body is totally co-extensive with our denser material body, and the two influence and exchange with each other, as would be expected from Relativity theory. We see that this energy body can be detected and unconsciously directed and altered.

11

The Science of Breath

Medical science has repeatedly shown how the mind affects the body. One way that body/mind interaction is mediated is through the breath. The breath can be both voluntary and involuntary, and "energy body" of the organism can be directly influenced by it. By executing a simple breathing exercise one can go beyond and get a direct experience of the energy body. Using the technique of slow diaphragmatic breathing and alternate nostril breathing as outlined ahead, one can begin to mildly experience the energy body in a relaxed state.

The Breathing Exercise

This technique is called in Sanskrit "Nadi shodhanam". Before starting be in a relax mode and do not get disturbed by telephone or any other environmental distractions. Then place yourself in a comfortable posture by sitting on the ground.

Your spine should be supported at the base and you should be sitting still. Bring your right hand to your nose with your index and middle fingers held down in such a way that the right thumb is used to close the right nostril and ring finger is used to close left nostril. With the right nostril closed by your right thumb, exhale completely through the left nostril. It is important that your exhalation be smooth, slow and deep. At the end of the exhalation phase, inhale slowly through the left nostril and fill the lungs. After full inhalation close the left nostril with the ring finger and exhale through the right nostril. After full exhalation, inhale through the right nostril and again close the right nostril, exhaling through the left nostril. The duration of inhalation and exhalation must be equal.

Continue to focus your attention only on the sound of the breath and either in the center of your chest or middle of the eyebrow. Repeat this pattern three or more times for full cycle of five complete breaths. When you have completed five full cycles, rest your attention at the root of your nose and breathe slowly. Your subjective state will be altered. You will see that breathing and consciousness are interrelated.

If your bio-gravitational or energy field were measured before and after this exercise, definite differences would be found. The accomplished yogi can slow his or her respiration to seventy six cycles per hour through what is called "*Ujjayi Pranayama*" and thereby deeply influence the subtle energy body.

The olfactory nerve responsible for the sense of smell is linked to the limbic system that is the base of our stratum of our emotionality.

It is found that this nerve has 1½ to 2½ hour cycle of either left or right nostril dominance. In other words, we breath primarily through the left nostril for 1½ hours or so, and then primarily through the right. Neurophysiologists have found that inhaling either clean air or air containing substances that can be detected through smell stimulates the olfactory nerve, which can affect emotion. This natural alternation of breath from nostril has been intimately associated with the brain function, ancient yogis discovered this, and it appears to affect the functioning of the left or right hemispheric modalities.

The breathing techniques described above are used to increase awareness and to control involuntary nervous system. The autonomic nervous system is divided into two areas, the sympathetic and the parasympathetic. The sympathetic nervous system governs more active, externally oriented system of the body. When this system is activated, the heart rate increases, adrenaline is secreted, and then the stress is developed.

The parasympathetic system governs more resting functions such as digestion, relaxation, etc.

An optimal balance between the two is essential for good health. Each inhalation stimulates the sympathetic system; each exhalation stimulates the parasympathetic system.

By slowly learning the breathing techniques the motion of lungs through the observation and control of the breath, you can also regulate the heart function. When the right nervous system is brought under control that portion of mind body is brought under control. There is also a direct line to the internal organs of the body through the right nerve. Thus, many functions of the autonomic nervous system can be controlled. This system is intimately related to the conscious control of the breath.

The yogis breathing of *pranayama* are a direct way to influence the 6,000 miles of nervous system within the adult human body. Through practice the 500 cc we regularly breath is greatly expanded in the full diaphragmic breath to 3000 cc. Think of it as primary energy exchange with the environment. We can survive for almost a week without water. We can survive a month without food. How many minutes do we have without oxygen ?

A certain state of consciousness associated with breathing techniques can subtly influence the areas of the body mind field. Simple diaphragmatic breathing and alternate nostril usage will induce a state of autonomic balance accompanied by calm and expansiveness along with the capacity to slow down the rate of thoughts.

Reflection solely on the breath flowing evenly at the root of the nose and relaxation of the body will lead to a pleasantly altered state of perception and experience.

12

Information and Transformation

Patanjali, Yoga said, "By perfectly concentrated meditation on mind/images is gained the understanding of thoughts of others. By perfectly concentrated meditation on sympathy, compassion and kindness is gained the power of interior union with others."

How does the information exchange between two yogis or two psyches take place. First they have to center themselves and should have loving relationship between them. The point of interaction includes both the other systems, and there is information exchange between psyches separated by space.

The Euclidean space between distant psyches is somehow bent, certainly altered, and the possibility therein exists for time to undergo a fundamental alteration. Space-time becomes fluid. The personal or individual unconscious is activated by the emotional energy of a powerful constellation of events, and those two people will have powerful thought transformations due to inner network.

These relationships, in turn, occur as a reflection of events occurring in the system of the collective unconscious of humanity at large. This is not to say that one system causes the events in the others. Rather, they occur simultaneously as a manifestation of ultimate interconnectedness. Energy and information are exchanged in a "supraliminal" way, which means moving faster than the speed of light. At the above the speed of light causality is radically transformed.

In order that information travels free the energy fields of the individuals involved must be harmonious, or in phase sequence. In other words, there needs to be coherence across and within the patterns. Intimate contact and emotional coherence where two people feel the same thing at the same time should exist.

It is to be noted that there are different levels of awareness for the observing ego. The autonomic nervous system also receives greater attention during sleep, and other senses of space and time categories are renegotiated. It is quite possible that some other center in the body such as the solar plexus (called by some other brain) affects consciousness and is implicated in the autonomic nervous system.

Psychodynamic theory explains the conscious, preconscious, and unconscious levels of the psyche's operation.

For information, to travel these various levels of consciousness and energy operative within and through the psyche need to come into phase coherence relationship with other psyches under specific condition outlined above.

At times the psyche appears to us to operate as an open field with networks of influence and mutual formation. In non-ego dominated conditions it "connects" with other psyches. It has a certain wave/field character at such times. At other times the psyche seems contracted and tensed. It is just like a discrete particle aspect of its character. The psyche, over duration and in different conditions, seems to expand and contract, and show the dual manifestation of particle and wave. It literally "pulses" at certain energy levels. Various members of the system appear to share these frequencies or energy levels which operate through and within each individual psyche.

When the energy of thought moves like a wave it absorbs much energy and they resonate and constantly interact with the other persons thought.

The interaction of electromagnetic radiations with matter is basically similar although different materials are affected at different wavelengths. The resonating structure thus determines the radiation which will affect it. We exist in a matrix of resonating frequencies and structure.

Know Yourself

Today the knowledge of different branches of science is expanding. Our knowledge of science gained in the past is being changed by new discoveries and more advancement of mind.

Generally in this world people want to gain knowledge of objects outside the body. The object comes to your mind through the faculty of knowledge. Suppose you look at a flower. Flower is an object. You notice the colour of the flower. You smell the flower. Your energy from your body emanates from your body and moves to the flower. There are three types of activities take place.

One is the flower, which is called known. Another is the subject, which is called the knower. Third is the knowledge, which is the knowledge gained in the process of learning of object? In the majority of cases the energy travels from knower to known. It is only one-directional energy. The arrow is pointing in one direction only. The knowledge of gaining flower is one direction only.

Now, imagine that the arrow is pointing in both the directions. The arrow emanating from the knower travels towards the flower or the object. Now imagine the arrow is moving towards the knower.

In this case, you will start gaining the knowledge of your body. You will find that you are quite different from the body. You will gain knowledge of your body. All the techniques of meditation are revealed to the knower. Lord Krishna said in the *Gita* that " This body, O son of Kunti, is called the field, and one who knows the field, and one who knows this body is called the knower of the field."

All the techniques of meditation are revealed the knower. Indian Yogis have said that self-remembering is very important in learning your body. They said that whenever you are knowing something always remember yourself. Your knowledge must be double-arrowed pointing in two directions. It must flow simultaneously in two directions—the known and the knower. This is called self-remembering.

Buddha called it *samyak smriti*—right-mindfulness. He said that your mind is not in a right mindfulness if it knows only one point. It must know both.

And then a miracle happens. If you are aware of both known and the knower, suddenly you become the third. You will find that how your body is different from your mind. You become the witness of both—object and the body. This becomes witness of your body and object is the important step of gaining peace and tranquility.

When you witness yourself you will find false ego, the ten senses and the brain, the five sense objects, desire, hatred, happiness, distress, the aggregate, the life symptoms, and convictions—all these are considered, in summary, to be the field of activities and its interactions within you.

If you completely detach yourself from the body and the object you will witness the activity of both of them. Once you know that, you will have become both. Then the rose—the known, and the knower—the mind, are just two wings of you. The object and subject are two wings of you and you are the center of both. They are extensions of yourself. Then the world and divine are both extension of you and you have come to the very center of being. And this center of being is just a witness.

13

Peace Through Heart Chakra

Heart is a place of great peace. It is believed that heart is the center of love and peace. If the *chakra* of the heart is developed it will fill you with emotions of love and peace within yourself.

In order to develop this *chakra* you have to be in perfect relaxed state. Forget about your worries and problems. Sit down in a comfortable position on bed or ground. Hook off your telephone. Think about your heart. Close your eyes and just feel the area between the two armpits. Bring your total attention on heart.

Forget all other parts of the body. Imagine that rays of white light are entering in your heart. Fix that light on your heart and relax you will be filled with peace and tranquility.

There are two areas in the body, particular centers where particular feelings can be created. These peaceful feelings can only be created in your heart. The heart radiates peace. That is why people all over the world without any distinction of caste, religion, country, educated or uneducated have felt this love. This love arises somewhere in the heart. No scientific explanation exists.

If you want to send love to someone then that will pose a little problem to yourself. You are making that person more important than yourself. You become a dependent on that person. This will give you peace sometime. If other person is thinking something else then you cannot have peace.

If that person is also sending the same force of love towards you then you are in perfect peace.

If you meditate in your heart by focussing a ray of light that will bring perfect peace and harmony. This peace not a single, lover will disturb you. The heart is naturally the source of peace, so you are not creating anything. You are simply coming to a source which is always there. And this imagination will help you become aware that heart is filled with peace.

Try this method : when you will be in peace between two armpits at the center of the heart the world will look illusory. This is a sign that you have entered meditation. The world looks like a dreamy, a dreamlike existence. It is there and world looks like a film of a projector. In this meditative criteria the world becomes unreal. You will feel bliss and peace.

This type of meditation is good at the time of sleep. At that time if you feel peace in heart then you will have peaceful sleep and you will not be disturbed by bad dreams. This is good for people who are suffering with insomnia—it helps deeply. If you feel that the world is unreal, tension dissolves. You will reach a deep stage of sleep. And in the morning you will feel fresh, so young, the whole energy vibrating and just coming from the center back to the circle.

If you feel peace and tranquility in heart everybody will behave differently with you. They will be more loving and more kind and less resistant to you. The magnet of peace in heart will attract more and more people. When you are disturbed that magnet becomes inactive, then you are not going to attract any one. You will repel everybody.

14

Good Eating Habits

Food intake plays an important role in getting power of mind. Medical science professor Dr. Rick Weindruch of Wisconsin-Madison said that "Secret to long life is eat less". Prof Nelson said that aging and old age is a byproduct of inactivity and poor nutrition. Good eating habits with moderate exercise will help in building healthy body and powerful mind.

Exercise builds muscles and burns fat, makes the heart and lungs work more efficiently, lowers the concentration of sugars circulating in the blood, increases the flow of thought provoking blood to the brain, and makes the bones stronger and more dense. Exercise also increases the body's metabolic rate, which will prevent declining of health. Some doctors had concluded that Oxygen is essential for animal life, but some oxygen becomes electrically charged, and they are called free radicals. Many experts believe that free radicals are to blame for much of the progressive physical and mental decline.

Eat vitamins E and C. These dietary supplements reduce the heart disease, cataracts, and skin changes can control these free radicals.

Longevity and good health according to Tom Johnson, the university of Colorado researched that age I in one of the genes in the group of 13,000 genes when mutated can greatly extend the life. This discovery gave credence to the notion that aging may be controlled by a molecular programme.

All these ageing and bad health problems can be reduced by taking balanced diet. In *Gita,* Krishna said that there are three types of foods one is foods of goodness, second food is food of passions and third is food of ignorance. Food of goodness produces good effect in the body and mind. Food of goodness comprises of fresh fruits, lightly cooked vegetables, whole bread, pasta, 1 per cent fat milk, high fibre breakfast cereals and curds.

Food of goodness will produce good results on the body and mind. Mind will not be distracted by sex. These food habits will help in concentration of mind and meditation.

Another type of food is food of passions. These foods are fully cooked eggs, chicken, red meats, fish and various other types of meat mixed with vegetables. Most of the people in the United States eat foods of passion. Due to increase of such type of food people are lazy, over-weight and indulge in sex. These types of food are full of fat and saturated fats. There are about 33 per cent people who are overweight and become victims of various diseases.

The third type of food is food of ignorance. This type of foods comprises uncooked meat, date expired foods, drinking alcohols and drugs. This type of food causes delusion in mind and causes mind to get panicked and people fall from grace of God. Most of the criminals eat these types of food and this helps them in committing crimes.

In culture of Western civilization people can't live without meats. So the best way of eating habits should be :

Gill rather than fry

Use lean meats, eat fish, beans, legumes, or nuts.

Eat low-fat cheese.

Use unsaturated oils for cooking, such as olive oil, and sunflower oils.

Avoid large quantities of high-fat foods, like, cakes, pastries, chips and chocolate.

Eat no more than four eggs a week.

Eat oily fish like tuna, salmon.

Reduce total sugar, use fruit rather than add sweetness, choose low sugar drinks.

Increase dietary fibre, and reduce salt.

Conclusion

Principal of Energization: Physical body is changing every day, every minute, every second. Doctors have found in eight year all the cells of the body are changed and we have completely changed. The nature of matter is change but nature of spirit is changelessness. Our cells are nothing but whiling motion electrons and protons whirling around the nucleus. Each molecules and atoms have space between them. It looks compact and sold due to high motion of electrons. In order to keep the activities of the bodily cells in motion certain external factors are necessary.

1. Sunshine and air
2. Oxygen
3. Food
4. Water or fruit juices.

But, more important the cells are also internally energized by our super consciousness. Without this vital force the external sources of bodily energy are of no avail in maintaining life in the body. Ordinarily, people eat lot of food in the United States. There are more than 60 per cent of the people are overweight and more than 30 per cent are obese. Result is there are suffering with diabetic, heartattack and high blood pressure. The realisation then comes that this body-battery must also be recharged by the inner source. Car needs a battery to run. In spite of all the components if battery is not there car will not run. Battery supplies the electric current to run the car. Similarly, our body car will not function by means of indirect outer sources, i.e., food, oxygen, liquids, air. But inner source of will, which causes vibrating life current from the invisible dynamo of Cosmic Energy to flow into the body through the medulla oblongata, the base of super consciousness. (The medulla is located at the base of the skull joins the neck.)

It is the vital life energy that converts oxygen, solids, and liquids of food into force that keeps us alive. When we put food into a stomach it must be converted into energy before it is use to the body. And when the energy is withdrawn, it is the life energy that forces the residue of this mass of waste material out of body through the pores, intestines, and kidneys. Of all the body parts the surgeon cannot operate only medulla oblongata. Why? Because it is the centre of all the centres of life in the brain and the spine. It is the centre through the life force enters the body. From this life force enters in brain, hearts and other chakras.

We can learn to live more and more by that eternal supply of cosmic energy, which is always present around us and we can recharge our bodies with vitality. We have to keep our body fit and healthy in order to progress in self-realisation. A body that is free from disease and weakness presents less resistance to the meditation methods and practices by which self-realisation is attained. Since it is difficult to concentrate and meditate while the aches and pains of the body continually have the attention of the mind. The path will easy if the imperfections of the body are eliminated and if the operation of its functions are so harmoniously arranged that mind need not at any time be interrupted in meditation because of the demands of the physical body.

By constantly doing meditation and enjoying the peaceful after effects of meditation in mind, discarding illusory changes and believing in external life and feeling the ocean of immortal bliss underlying the changeable waves of experiences we can bring about not only the perpetually youthful consciousness of the soul, but also maintain youthfulness of body, if so desired. When the body is found to be, not isolated from spirit, but number of falling waves of vibrating currents in the ocean of Cosmic Consciousness, we may implant in the body the perpetually rejuvenating power of spirit.

So long we dwell in the material plane we cannot encompass the super consciousness no matter how desirous it may be doing so. By practice of the scientific concentration and meditation techniques taught in the previous chapters the sincere student can increase and refine the receptivity of his consciousness so that he may ultimately perceive the super consciousness present in every atom of creation. By intuitive practice man becomes aware of his oneness with the super consciousness. This man then enjoys all the bliss of the bounty nature. Self-realisation and chakras faithfully practiced will be found to be sure and effective combatant against bodily diseases and inharmonious conditions of the mind.

The Dynamic Power of Will: Strong will is the powerful dynamo, which pumps the power in our mind to accomplish some desired result. Without the strong will power we cannot do any adventures action. Wish is a week or helpless desire of the mind. Desire is the little strong wish. An intention is little more powerful than desire. This intention also ends up in frustration if we did not get success after our best attempt. When this intention becomes very powerful then it is called will power. Will power and act until victory is achieved no matter how impossible of accomplishment his goal may seem.

Blind Will: If the will is not guided by wisdom then it is called blind will. Most young people use this explosive blind will without any worthwhile purpose, wasting energy and higher possibilities on passions, temptations, fast driving, rash resolutions, ungoverned appetites, and so forth. It is just like a bee for love for fragrance sits on a lotus flower, the petals entomb it if the bee forgets to get out before they close. The moose loves music and is lured to death by the flute of the hunter. So each of these creatures dies because they addicted to a single sense. But man is attached to all five senses, and he must watch his step if he would save himself from his blind will, which urges him to jump into one of the trap of the five senses lures. Any will, which is not guided by discrimination, is bound to failure. But if one's thinking will retain its power if discrimination is used and unselfish will and resolve around a definite purpose, it becomes "dynamic will". When such will be used for wholesome purposes and actions are in tune with universal harmony or good the will is strengthened and leads to success. A wrongly used will weakens itself, owing to lack of encouragement from truth, as it's out of tune with the universal order. When one knows that his objectifies is worthwhile, then the tenacity of his will becomes greater.

The man of will power will say, "I will use my dynamic power of will to fight for the truth until success comes. If death intervenes I shall take up my activity with renewed determination in another incarnation, until I have fulfilled my good purposes."

A strong will by its own dynamic force creates a way of fulfillment of its intentions. By its very strength, the will sets into motion certain vibrations in the atmosphere, and nature, with its law of order, system, and efficiency, its greatest strength from an honest purpose, lofty motives and a noble solicitude for doing good to the world at large. A stong will is never going in vain. God did not make us like a robot, it given us a free will. God' desire is to use our free will without whim or temptation. His will is guided by wisdom. To teach people not to use wisdom is not only ridiculous denial of Divine wish Temptation is delusive, compelling, conflicting, joy-expecting thought which should used to pursue happiness-making truth and not misery-producing error. Although God is the creator of consciousness, the vitiated consciousness in man turns away from him and tries to lure the soul to concentrate upon temporary pleasures of the senses.

Some Western athletes have learned to control certain muscles by will, but failed to see the scientific principles underlying such control. The yogis of India have a large number of postures that they practice in order to strengthen and develop their will power. The will can be utilised to develop the body: and the will itself is developed in the process by the very exercising of it.

You cannot get the answer from the supersoul just in one or two attempts. You cannot get an answer by just calling someone and then running away. Continuously do yoga and payer to God through your calm mental microphone until you hear his answering voice.

Divine will has no boundaries: The only savior of man is a constantly progressive dynamic will. Human will, however powerful, is still limited by the circumference of the body and body of the physical universe. Whereas divine will has no boundaries it works in all bodies, in all things. When by deep meditation and by wisdom-guided, unflinching, never discouraged determination we can successfully keep our will revolving around all our noble desires, then our will becomes one with divine will.

For absolute control of your life and for destroying prenatal and postnatal root-causes of failure, you must exercise your will in every undertaking, until it shakes off its mortal delusion of being human will and becomes all powerful divine will.

Communication

The message you communicate with an another human being has nothing to do with what you say, it has nothing to do with the look on the vibrations of your face, it's much deeper than that much deeper!

It's the vibrations that emanate from you, if your vibrations are paranoid that's what's being received.

And you realise that every moment you are a full statement of your being, and you are sending out vibrations that are affecting everything around you, which in turn is affecting everything that comes back. If your selfish ego is under control and your mind is open to receive all spiritual vibrations you will receive many powerful vibrations that will change your thinking and pumps energy that will help you in advancement in inward journey.

Love has to spring spontaneously from within: And it is no way amenable to any form of inner or outer force. Love and coercion can never go together; Though love cannot be forced but it can be awakened in him, through love awakening you can change the mind of any one. Criminals are changed to good person.

Love is unconquerable and irresistible; and it goes on gathering power and spreading itself, until eventually it transforms everyone whom it touches. (Meher Baba)

Buddha said that Watch your speech, Watch your thought, Watch your calmness. Get your calm centre going. Living your life in such a way as to get yourself straight; to get free of attachment that just keeps sucking you in all the time. This will keep our life straight.

Do your work without attachment. If you are attached then your action will be bounded and did not get you out from birth and death cycle. Do everything you want to do with full sincerity and unattached.

Sadhana

This sadhana will help us to get rid of my ego. If I get free of my ego we will get free of our ego. We are all the same being and we move fast if we all move together fast. This will help us to great stride in evaluation.

Just work on your self by doing meditation. Everything you work on yourself, you get calmer you hear more and sense more you are more present. Your outlook will be widen. You will get sense of enjoyment within self. Your power of perception will increase.

Trust the messages coming from your heart and intuition. This journey is an inner journey. The charisma of an impure being such as Hitler would not be of influenced on another person were that person totally honest with himself and totally true to inner voice.

Short Cut Way for Sadhana

1. Close your left nostril by right hand, take three deep breaths out of your right nostril, then eject it after 20 seconds by left nostril and assuming that dark red air which is all the bodily disease. Do this practice 10 times.

2. Close your right nostril. Now deep breath three times by left nostril, then eject it after 20 seconds and assuming as blue-gray which is all your mental obstacles and anger.

3. Now visualise that white sun light is entering on ajna (the point between the eyebrows) then meditate that white light for 10 minutes it help you in opening your third eye and help you in getting rid of sins and wrong.

4. Now, visualise a red beam light entering the throat chakra a middle point of throat Hold that light 10 minutes. This beams rids you of lapses of speech of harsh and untruth sound.

5. Now, visualise a blue beam of light coming to your heart and hold your visualisation for 10 minutes. This will empower

the power of love. Also helps you to get rid of bad thought of your heart, this also helps you in keeping your heart stronger.

Take four promises:

1. I will become enlightened for benefit of mankind.
2. I will the roots of all delusive passions.
3. I will follow the true religion of mankind.
4. I will try to love all mankinds and avoid violence.

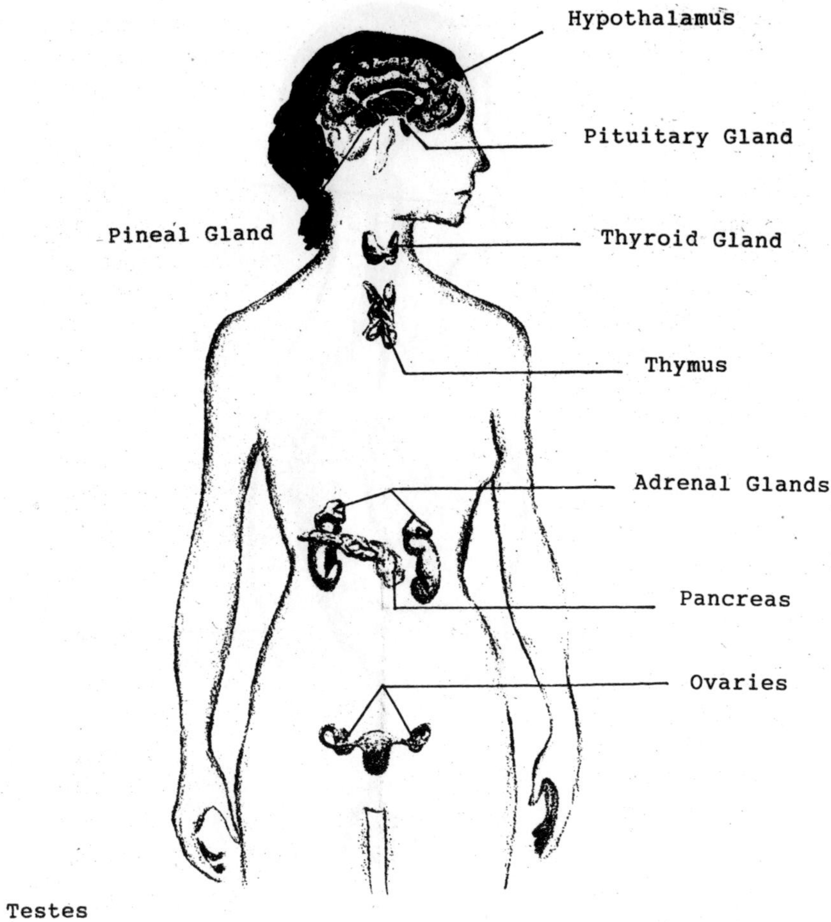

Control Centers

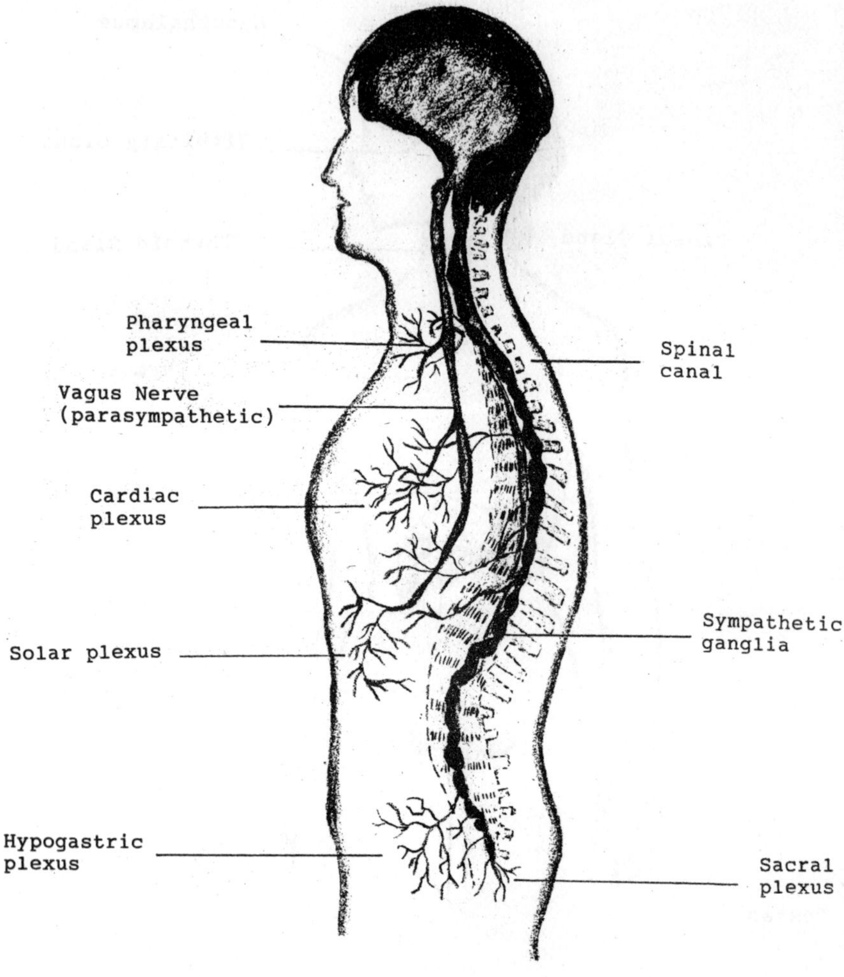

Autonomic Nervous System
and Plexuses

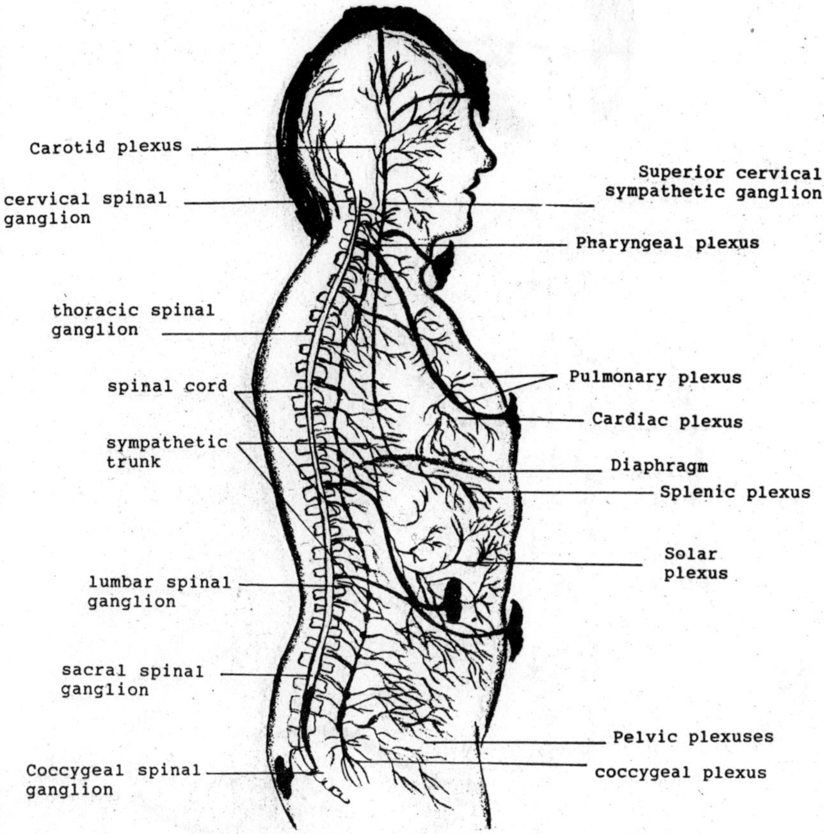

The Chakras and the Nervous System

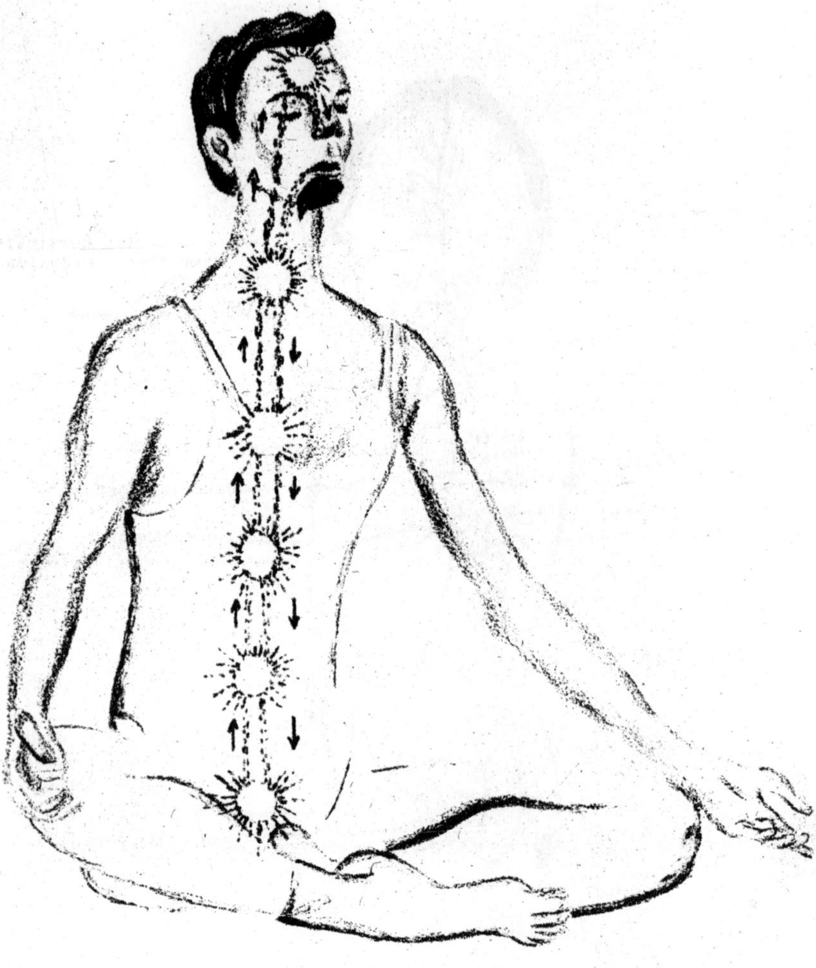

ENERGY CENTERS

CHAKRA EXERCISE

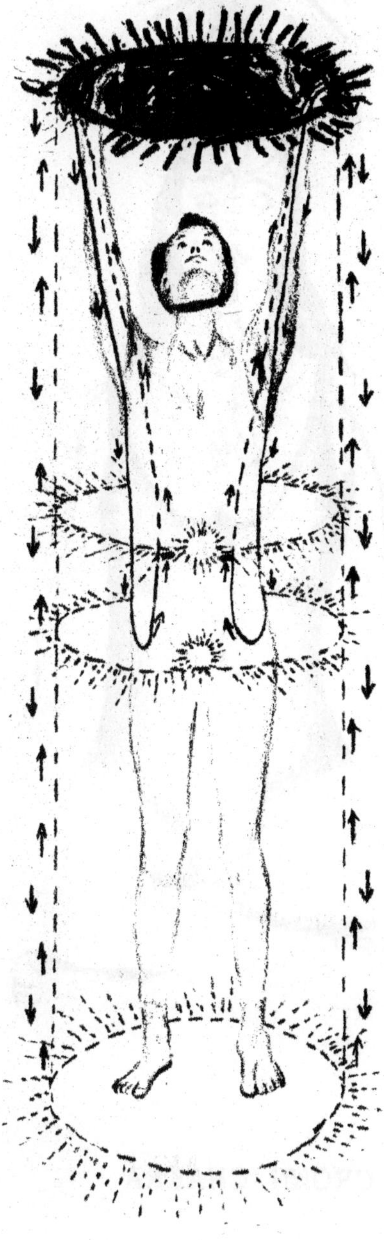

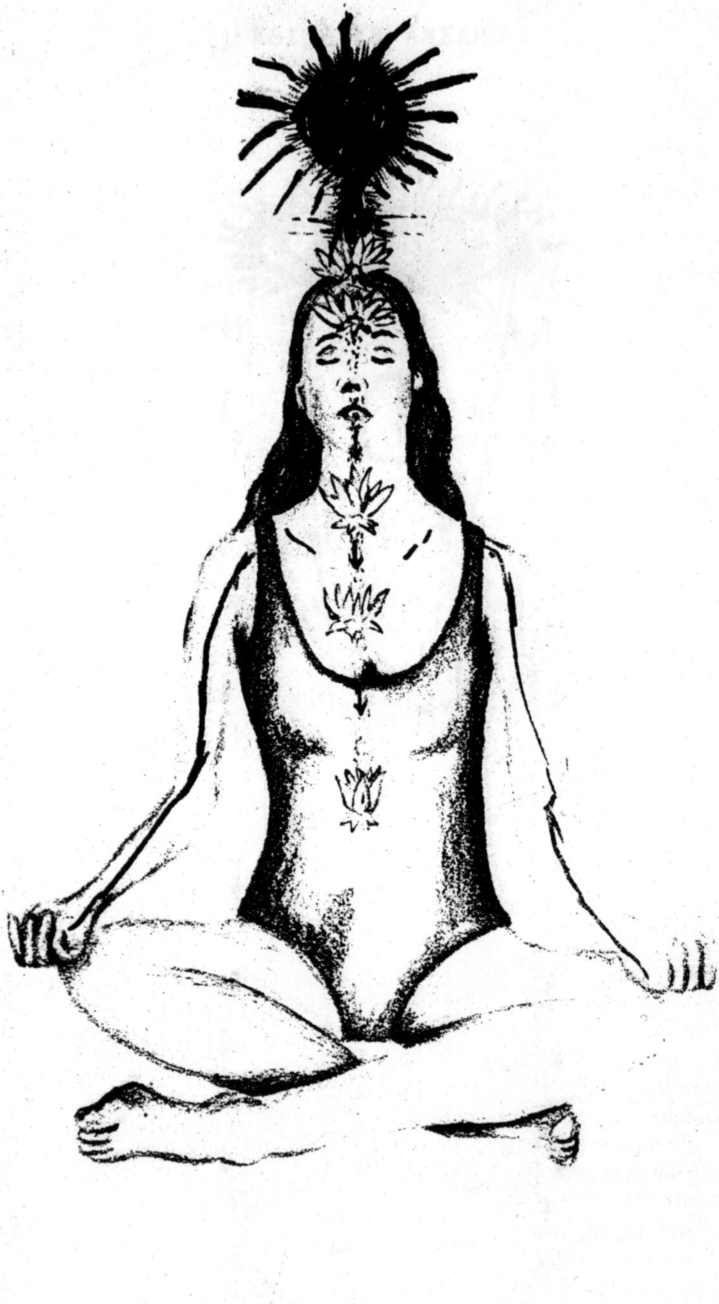

CROWN CHAKRA

Index